Ethnomedicine

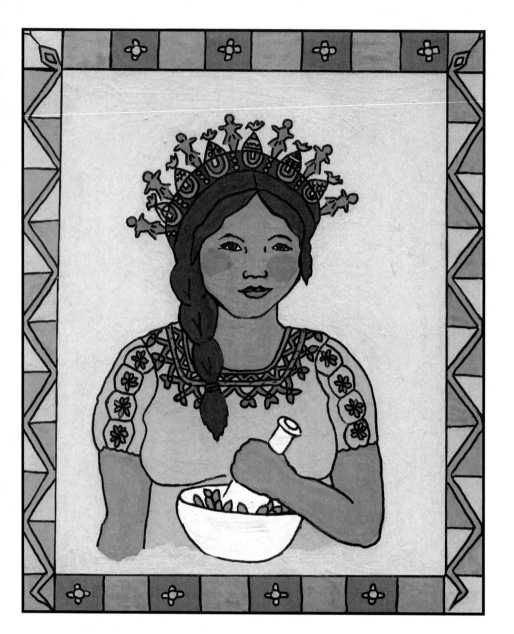

Ethnomedicine

Pamela I. Erickson
University of Connecticut

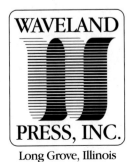

WAVELAND
PRESS, INC.
Long Grove, Illinois

For information about this book, contact:
    Waveland Press, Inc.
    4180 IL Route 83, Suite 101
    Long Grove, Illinois 60047-9580
    (847) 634-0081
    info@ waveland.com
    www.waveland.com

Cover Photo: Pamela Erickson, statue of medicine Buddha at
Binglingsi Thousand Buddha Caves, Gansu Province, China.

Frontispiece: Artist Bonnie Atwood is a freelance illustrator
whose work can be found at www.owlfoot.com

Contents

5   The Healing Lessons of Ethnomedicine   99

Acknowledgments

There are so many people who deserve thanks for seeing me through this book—Louise Badiane, Nanette Barkey, Steve Beckerman, Merrill Eisenberg, Vicki Erickson, Celia Kaplan, Mark Macauda, Sheryl Rosenthal, and Merrill Singer for moral support; Marsha Quinlan, Merrill Singer, and the anonymous reviewer for editorial and content suggestions, most especially Marsha Quinlan for her extensive, thoughtful review and the many suggestions that were incorporated; Pat Townsend and Ann McElroy for suggesting I write this book in the first place—they, along with Susan Scrimshaw, are my three incredible mentors; Bonnie Atwood, Dexter and Atticus Lazenby, and Jacob Murrow—for general whimsy, artistic insight, music, and kayak/canoe breaks; Bonnie Atwood for her marvelous illustration, the frontispiece; and every single student who ever took my ethnomedicine class. The resulting book is both more and less than I envisioned, as teaching and writing are always creative learning processes that lead you to their own ends. Thank you all!

Chapter 1

What Is Ethnomedicine?

The term ethnomedicine sounds exotic to most people. It implies something other than biomedicine—something more ethnic, less scientific, and more magical. Ethno means race, people, or cultural group. Ethnomedicine is simply the study of the medical systems or healing practices of a cultural group, the cross-cultural comparison of such systems, and increasingly the study of the multiple use of different medical therapies. For medical anthropologists, it also encompasses the domains of individual experience, discourse, knowledge, practice, and meaning; the social, political, and economic relations of health; the ecology of health and illness; and the interpretation of human suffering and health concerns in space and time (Baer et al. 2003, Lock and Scheper-Hughes 1996, McElroy and Townsend 2004, Nichter 1992, Sargent and Johnson 1996, Scheper-Hughes and Lock 1987).

Although the study of ethnomedicine has been the province of medical anthropology, this book is not about medical anthropology and its theories and methods. Rather its purpose is to provide a broad understanding of the basic organizing principles that underlie all medical systems, the full range of theories of disease causation, their geographical distribution, and the historical trends that led to biomedical dominance. It is intended as a primer on ethnomedicine that will illustrate cross-cultural concepts of illness and healing and relate them to our Western, biomedical understanding of disease, curing, and efficacy. Only by understanding this broader picture can we fully understand the nature of healing and the current worldwide trend toward use of multiple medical systems and therapies.

This chapter discusses how ethnomedicine is conceptualized within anthropology and how biomedicine has changed from excluding

1

to incorporating alternative medicines. Then an outline of the major
components of all medical systems is presented to provide the foundation for understanding illness and healing as individual biological and
social processes.

ANTHROPOLOGY AND ETHNOMEDICINE

W. H. R. Rivers (1924) launched the study of ethnomedicine in
anthropology by treating medical systems as social institutions and
suggesting that seemingly implausible curing practices were rational
when viewed from the perspective of indigenous disease theories. He
also linked ethnomedicine to magic and religion, a stereotype that per-
vaded the field for half a century. As a result, ethnomedicine began as
the study of "beliefs and practices relating to disease which are the
products of indigenous cultural development and are not explicitly
derived from the conceptual framework of modern medicine" (Hughes
1968, cited in Foster and Anderson 1978:5).

Defining ethnomedicine as what biomedicine is not, however,
lumps together a dizzying array of medical systems that vary widely in
the extent to which they are codified (have a written tradition), orthodox (accepted as doctrine), legitimate (upheld by law), and effective
(usually measured by biomedical standards). Thus, American chiropractic, Traditional Chinese medicine (TCM), and Indian Ayurvedic
medicine, all of which have a long history, a written tradition, medical
schools, and legal standing in the countries in which they originated,
are lumped in the same category with the myriad, largely oral, herbal
traditions throughout the world and with spiritual healing traditions,
such as faith healing, voodoo, and shamanism. The only thing they all
have in common is that they do not use the techniques of biomedicine
to heal and they are not based on the scientific materialism that guides
biomedicine, namely experiment and statistical validation of assump-
tions and the breaking down of complex phenomena into component
parts (e.g., the various organ systems of the body) each of which is dealt
with by itself (scientific reductionism).

Excluding biomedicine from the study of medical systems hin-
dered the ability of anthropologists (and others) to think about and
understand how different medical systems effect healing while using
widely different techniques and encouraged study of ethnomedical systems as discrete, internally consistent entities. Yet this separation was
understandable considering the staggering advances that had been
made in medical science in the 20th century (e.g., immunization, antibiotics, anesthesia, genetics), surgical techniques, biomedical technology, and pharmaceutical development and those of public health in

infectious disease control, hygiene, and nutrition. Indeed, in the face of such triumphs, it was easy to forget that "until the beginning of the 19th century all medical practice was what we now call traditional" (Bannerman et al. 1983:11). Until the 1970s, biomedicine was the premiere medical system in the West and was dominant in world health considerations (Basch 1999, Magner 2005, Starr 1982). But, the success of biomedicine in treating the physical body forced it to hive off the psychological, social, spiritual, economic, and political from its purview of interest. Biomedicine focused on the physical body of the individual patient and the physical cause of his/her disease instead, paying little attention to the social context or the lived experience of the patient. This was a significant departure from its historical roots in Greco-Roman medicine, which were much more holistic and intuitive, as were other medical systems as well.

Nevertheless, the spectacular success of biomedicine and the ability of the West to dominate the rest of the world for most of the 20th century, first through colonialism and then through globalization and the domination of world markets and information systems, resulted in the hegemony of biomedicine worldwide (Baer et al. 2003). For almost a century, biomedicine has been the standard to which all other forms of healing have been compared.

Yet, even as the successes of biomedicine were noted, so too were its less spectacular results with chronic and degenerative diseases, which were becoming ever more important worldwide, following on the heels of the demographic transition that resulted in an aging and longer-lived population.[1] The first nail in the coffin of biomedical dominance came in 1978 when the World Health Organization (WHO) made the pivotal decision to include and promote traditional medicine in the delivery of primary health care to the world's populations (Bannerman et al. 1983, World Health Organization 1978). The second nail was the soaring cost of biomedical health care since the 1980s. The third nail was the erosion of faith in scientific medicine and increasing interest in other healing traditions spurred by greater access to health information on the Internet and consumers' desire to have more control over medical decision making (Jonas 2000, Fox 1997, Starr 1982). As a result, Western societies began to incorporate alternative healing systems into biomedicine just as non-Western societies had incorporated biomedicine into their traditional healing systems (Bannerman et al. 1983, Basch 1999, Young and Garro 1994/1981).

While these broad social changes were occurring, the discipline of anthropology was changing as well. Anthropologists began to question both the exclusion of biomedicine from the field of ethnomedicine and the dominance of biomedicine itself (Baer et al. 2003, Nichter 1992). Medical anthropology emerged as a distinct subdiscipline defined as "the cross-cultural study of medical systems and . . . the bioecological and sociocultural factors that influence the incidence of health and disease now and throughout human history" (Foster and Anderson 1978:1). This subtle shift allowed biomedicine, the West's ethnomedicine, to be included within the purview of ethnomedical studies (Hahn 1983). For most medical anthropologists, biomedicine is now considered only one of many medical systems that can be studied, like all the others, as a culturally embedded social institution to which various theoretical perspectives can be applied (Nichter 1992). Interdisciplinary interactions between anthropology, medicine, and public health within the context of national and international health initiatives[2] have fostered new ways of thinking about culture and health that evolved into the current emphasis on the delivery of culturally appropriate health care in nations with increasingly diverse populations.[3]

All of these developments resulted in a sea change for biomedical dominance. Yet, a basic tension between biomedicine and other medical traditions persists everywhere that biomedicine exists. It is undeniable that alternative therapies have become accepted by consumers of medical care in the West. In 1997, 42 percent of Americans used some form of alternative medicine (Eisenberg et al. 1998). In the industrialized countries, 20 to 65 percent of adults have used some kind of nonbiomedical therapy (Ernst 2000). There is also increasing recognition of alternative medicine by the scientific and biomedical communities (Eisenberg et al. 1998, Jonas 2000, Kelner and Wellman 2000, Sharma 1992). The many terms previously used to refer to nonbiomedical healing systems—indigenous, alternative, unorthodox, folk, ethnic, fringe, traditional, unofficial—highlighted their difference from biomedicine and often implied their inferiority (Bannerman et al. 1983, O'Connor 1995, Baer 2001). The current appellation, complementary and alternative medicine (CAM),[4] indicates the profound social changes that have begun to integrate nonbiomedical healing into health care in the West. However, CAM is still defined as what conventional medicine is not, and biomedicine tends to view CAM as separate and subordinate rather than truly integrative (Baer 2004). In addition, not all nonbiomedical therapies are included in CAM and what is included changes over time.

Even though there is still tension between biomedicine and CAM, it is agreed that "complementary and alternative medicine is here to stay. It is no longer an option to ignore it or treat it as something outside the normal processes of science and medicine" (Jonas 2000:xiv–xv). In the 21st century the West has begun a process of the scientifically based integration of CAM into the Western biomedical system. Studies of the efficacy of many CAM therapies are underway and there is already evidence that some CAM therapies are effective.[5] As such studies progress, however, we are wise to remember that there is no scientific evidence for the efficacy of many conventional biomedical therapies (Berman et al. 2000).

MEDICAL SYSTEMS

* medical systems as cultural performance?

According to George Foster, all human communities have responded to the threat of disease by developing a medical system, "the pattern of social institutions and cultural traditions that evolves from deliberate behavior to enhance health" (1983:17).[6] All medical systems are an integral part of the culture in which they developed, exist, and continue to evolve, and they cannot be understood apart from the social, religious, economic, and political organization of the societies in which they are found. They have both a cultural (shared modes of perception and behavior) and a social (roles and organization) aspect (Helman 2000, Landy 1977). Thus, medical systems are an integral part of the social organization of a community and they reflect the dominant cultural themes of society. For example, biomedicine in the United States is organized around the scientific methods and principles that underlie our rationalist approach to the world. It is a hierarchical system with physicians and hospital-based medicine at the top of the hierarchy. All other allied health professionals (e.g., nurses, occupational therapists, etc.) and out-of-hospital sources of care (e.g., clinics, rehabilitation centers, etc.) are secondary, however important they are in number and function. They are often subject to decisions made at the top level by physicians and hospital administrators. Except for the military, which has socialized medicine, health care is organized on a capitalist model. Finally, priority is given to the individual and his/her illness rather than the social context of ill health (e.g., family, environment, racism, poverty, etc.) and the role it may play in the causation or exacerbation of illness. In these ways, our medical system reflects our core cultural themes of independence, individualism, scientific positivism, and capitalism. In most, perhaps all, societies the threat of illness plays a powerful role in the moral order, and the threat of illness as an outcome of personal behavior is a powerful motivation to obey moral, social, and environmental norms. In Western culture and its medical system, personal responsibility for health is a paramount theme, and those who "choose" lifestyles that lead to illness are held responsible for those illnesses.

Components of Medical Systems

All medical systems share a set of basic components. Each system has a *theory of disease causation* that explains why people become ill. These causal theories provide the rationale for the treatment and prevention of illness and disease. Thus, all medical systems have both *preventive and curative strategies*. They also have *health care practitioners with specialized knowledge, skills, and training* who are recognized as healers through certification, examination, initiation, or public recognition. In some medical systems, training is codified (e.g., books, schools, licensing), in others it is informal (e.g., apprenticeship, self-taught, gift from higher powers). Theories of disease causation can range from elaborate, text-based, canons to oral traditions and folk narratives. Healers in all medical systems believe in their ability to heal, as do the people they treat. Attitudes toward healers are often ambivalent, however, because the power to cure implies its converse, the power to harm. Thus, healers often play powerful roles in their communities. Medical systems also *provide an organizational system for caring for the ill* that usually includes special places people go when they are sick, rules for interacting with healers, and defined roles for both patient and healer. Finally, there is a *system for paying the healer* for his or her services. Payment can be either monetary or in-kind (e.g., exchange of goods and services).

Sectors of Health Care

In complex societies, it is useful to think of medical systems in terms of three sectors of health care (Helman 2000, Kleinman 1980)—the popular sector, the professional sector, and the folk sector. The *popular sector* is nonprofessional. It includes the individual and his/her social network—family, friends, neighbors, coworkers, church communities, self-help groups, and discussions with people who have special experience with a particular health problem (e.g., an uncle who has diabetes or a grandmother who knows herbal remedies for children's stomach upsets). The popular sector is where illness is first recognized and where the quest for treatment begins. Within the family, women are usually the primary providers of health care for both children and adults. Treatment includes self-medication, over-the-counter medications, herbal remedies, and other nonprofessional healing therapies (e.g., diet, lifestyle change, spiritual). Prevention consists of maintaining culturally agreed upon guidelines for health maintenance with respect to lifestyle (e.g., diet, exercise, sleep, dress, work, and good conduct). Worldwide it is estimated that 70 to 90 percent of all health care takes place in this sector (Helman 2000, Kleinman et al. 1978). This sector is the least organized of the three and lacks some of the components of an organized medical system, most notably training and payment of providers; yet the way care is managed in this sector reflects the dominant theories of disease causation and treatment in a society, and it is the point of origin for health seeking behavior in the professional and folk sectors, both of which exhibit all the components of a medical system.

The *professional sector* includes the organized, legal healing professions (e.g., physicians, dentists) and recognized paramedical professions (e.g., nurses, physical therapists, chiropractors, etc.) in a society—for example, biomedicine and osteopathy in United States; Ayurvedic, Unani, and biomedicine in India; and Traditional Chinese medicine and biomedicine in China. The professional sector is also home to some of the healing strategies that are subordinate but complementary to biomedicine such as acupuncture and homeopathy in the United States. Biomedicine is firmly established throughout most of the world today, due in large part to the work of the World Health Organization and to the continued support of biomedicine in unilateral and multilateral aid programs from the developed to the less-developed countries, as well as the general dominance of Western economies and technologies in the world. However, access to biomedical care is uneven in less-developed countries, often existing only in urban areas. This has been exacerbated by the soaring cost of biomedical care over the last three decades that has been propelled by the development of expensive technologies, therapies, and pharmaceuticals. Today, biomedical care is financially out of reach for most people in the less-developed countries and for many people in the developed countries as well (e.g., the 45 million Americans, 15.6% of the population, without health insurance [DeNavas-Walt et al. 2005]). The increasing cost of biomedicine and the realization that biomedical services would probably never be available on a routine basis to most of the world' s population led to the change in policy at WHO to focus on primary health care and to promote both biomedicine and traditional medicine.

The folk sector includes both sacred and secular healers who are not part of the professional medical system. These healers are more specialized than individuals in the popular sector, but they are usually not recognized by the professional sector. Thus, they operate between the popular and professional sectors of health care. There are many kinds of folk healers, and they range from healers who have secular, technical expertise like lay midwives, bonesetters, and herbalists who are found in most societies of the world to more specialized spiritual healers (e.g., shamans, witches, faith healers) whose presence may be less widespread (Foster 1983). Their selection and training come from one or more of the following paths: inheritance (born into a family of healers), revelation (discovering a gift of healing), apprenticeship to another healer, and self-teaching. These healers are usually part of the communities in which they live and share the same basic cultural values as others in their community. Their healing techniques often involve a more holistic approach that restores social, environmental, and spiritual harmony as well as alleviation of illness for the individual. The folk sector has been the traditional object of ethnomedical study for anthropologists, although studies of the other two sectors are now extensive. It is also home to the healing traditions encompassed by CAM and to the many other indigenous healing systems that are not included in CAM but form part of what WHO calls traditional medicine.

Patients access and use these three sectors of health care in different ways. When a person feels sick or out of sorts, care is usually sought in the popular sector first. Often this is the only sector used for the many acute but non-life-threatening illnesses to which human beings fall victim. Indeed, the "80% Rule" tells us that four out of five people who seek medical care get better regardless of their treatment actions, indicating the powerful and natural tendency of the body to heal itself (Jonas 2000, Macdonald 2005, Thomas 1994). A person with a cold, for example, will be treated with home remedies (e.g., herbal tea, chicken soup, orange juice, rest) and perhaps some over-the-counter medications and herbal medicines (e.g., Tylenol, cough syrup, Echinacea). If home treatment fails to alleviate the complaint, however, and the illness is perceived to be worsening or more serious than first thought, some kind of professional advice will be sought and the patient will try another sector. For example, the cold may turn into bronchitis and the patient or his/her caregiver might seek biomedical care in the professional sector where the patient will be diagnosed and provided with antibiotics to cure the bronchial infection. Simultaneously, care might be sought in the folk sector for spiritual needs, and this is especially true when the illness becomes serious. If the patient's condition worsens to pneumonia and he/she has to be hospitalized, the family or a wider set of significant others—the sufferer's "therapy management group" (Janzen 1978)—might activate a prayer circle from their church to send healing energy to the patient. Alternatively, help might be sought in the folk sector from another kind of spiritual healer who can divine why the person has become sick and who can intervene in the spiritual world to put things right, or from a CAM provider, perhaps an acupuncturist who will assess the best points to needle to alleviate the lung congestion associated with bronchitis or pneumonia. As the professional and/or folk sectors are accessed, of course, the patient is likely to continue self-care initiated in the popular sector.

As this example shows, the different sectors of care can be used exclusively, sequentially, simultaneously, or repeatedly. There is rarely any coordination among health care providers when patients use multiple sectors, and healers from any sector often operate without knowledge of the other therapies that their patients might be using. This is especially true in the West where 72 percent of patients who use CAM do not tell their physician they do so (Eisenberg et al. 1998). The potential dangers of multiple therapies and medications for the patient have been cited repeatedly as a serious risk of CAM use by Western patients. Since health care is initiated and coordinated by the individual patient, the three sectors of care may only overlap at the level of the individual patient, resulting in a unique health care seeking and therapeutic trajectory for each patient.

HEALTH: DISEASE AND CURING, ILLNESS AND HEALING

As the old saying goes, "In this world nothing is certain but death and taxes." (Benjamin Franklin). To these I would add disease, injury, and accidents. None of us gets through life without at least a minor bout with illness (colds, flu), injury (cut finger, stubbed toe), and accident (falls, bumped head), and many, perhaps most of us, must face serious illness (heart disease, cancer, diabetes), injury (trauma), or accident (automobile, sports, or work related). If we are lucky enough to escape ourselves, we often become caregivers for others who are afflicted—our children, partners, siblings, friends, parents, grandparents, and others. Thus, *disease* and *illness* affect us all, but what do we really mean by these words? What do we mean by health?

According to Blaxter (2004) the medical model regards health as the absence of disease and the normal functioning of the body. The social model of health, however, suggests that health is something more than just the absence of disease or physical and mental impairment. Health implies a sense of wholeness, wellness, and well-being captured in the 1948 WHO definition: "a state of complete physical, mental and social well-being, and not merely the absence of disease or infirmity" (p. 19).

In the West, we have come to use the terms disease/curing and illness/healing in related but different ways. Disease is the medically defined, objective pathology afflicting the patient (e.g., malaria, cancer, PTSD). Sickness is the social manifestation of the body's physical reaction to a disease (e.g., fever, pain, rashes) that entitles the person to take on the socially defined sick role (Parsons 1951). Illness is the subjective experience of disease, sickness, or simply feeling that something is not right whether or not there is a diagnosis of disease (Eisenberg 1977, Hahn and Kleinman 1983, Kleinman 1980, Young 1982). Thus, as these terms are used technically in the health and social sciences, people can be sick (diagnosed with disease or risk factors for future disease such as hypertension or pre-diabetes) without being ill, and they can be ill (feel that something is wrong with them) without being sick. While most diseases and the symptoms and bodily processes they cause are thought to be relatively consistent across the individual biological bodies they afflict,[8] illness can be interpreted and reinterpreted by the individual, his/her family, and the wider community over time.

Just as we have set up a dichotomy between the objective reality of disease and the subjective experience of illness, we use the words curing to refer to the removal or correction of organic pathology and healing to refer to the broader experience of the restoration of physical, mental, emotional, social, and spiritual health (McGuire 1988,

O'Connor 1995). Just as we can have disease without illness and illness without disease, we can have curing without healing and healing without curing. A person afflicted with inoperable cancer can be healed if s/he comes to terms with her/his disease and *feels* a sense of peace and acceptance. Some AIDS patients, for example, report feeling far better after being diagnosed than before when they felt their lives were out of control and they lacked direction (Mosack et al. 2005). Alternatively, a woman recovering from knife wounds inflicted by her partner during a domestic violence incident can be cured in her body, but may never feel truly healed.

Disease/illness and curing/healing, of course, represent the classic Western body/mind dualism that pervades our notions of health. Biomedicine tends to focus on the physical, bodily problems of its patients, and thus, effecting a cure and/or maximizing physical function are the primary measures of success. To understand illness and healing, however, we must go beyond the physical body and understand these processes from the patient's perspective. Many indigenous, traditional, and CAM therapies are theoretically attuned to the broader notion of health that is implied in the term *healing*. For this reason they appeal to patients seeking a more philosophical or cosmological answer to the questions: Why me? Why now? What did I do to deserve this? How can I restore my health?

CONCLUSION

When faced with disease or illness, people turn to their medical system for help. Although the theories of disease causation and treatment strategies vary across different medical systems and often contradict one another, the goal of all medical systems is to provide people with a coherent way to understand their illness, a plan to restore their health, and a means to reintegrate them as functioning members of their communities.

In the following chapters we will explore the range of theories of disease causation that are known from biomedical and nonbiomedical systems. Chapter 2 contains an overview of human subsistence systems and how they have shaped health and disease; a discussion of the great medical traditions of ancient Greece, Rome, and Persia and their contribution to the development of biomedicine in the West; as well as the great medical traditions of India (Ayurvedic medicine), China (Traditional Chinese medicine), and Islamic medicine, all three of which, along with biomedicine, form the four major medical systems of the world today. These four medical traditions have affected local ethnomedical systems and each other over space and time just as they influence each other today. Chapter 3 contains a discussion of the range of theories of disease causation from complementary and alternative medicines that are not part of the great medical traditions. Chapter 4 looks at the geographical distribution of generalized patterns of theories of disease causation that tend to characterize the medical systems of broad cultural areas. The final chapter turns to a discussion of globalization, medical pluralism, and the search for healing in a complex world.

Knowledge of the basic tenets of the great medical traditions and the range of ethnomedical theory and practice beyond these great traditions provides the foundation that is essential for understanding why healing can and does occur within many, indeed probably all, medical systems. Knowledge of the broad cultural patterning of theories of disease causation provides a foundation for understanding the main issues involved in the provision of culturally appropriate health care. Finally, grounding the search for health and healing in the context of globalization allows us to understand the trend toward medical pluralism within an increasingly capitalist-driven, individualistic world medical system.

Notes

[1] This change in primary cause of morbidity and mortality from infectious to chronic diseases is known as the epidemiological transition (Omran 1971).

[2] The World Health Organization (WHO) has been instrumental in the worldwide spread of biomedicine since World War II to improve health in the developing countries.

[3] For more information, see the Office of Minority Health web page, http://www.omhrc.gov/clas/

[4] The National Center for Complementary and Alternative Medicine (NCCAM) in Washington, D.C. uses CAM as the official term for "a group of diverse medical and health care systems, practices, and products that are not presently considered to be part of conventional medicine." Complementary medicine is used with conventional medicine and alternative medicine is used instead of it.

[5] For example see Koenig et al. 1999, Lewis and Elvin-Lewis 2003, Sierpina and Frenkel 2005, and the more generally the *Journal of Scientific Review of Alternative Medicine*, http://www.sram.org/ (accessed 9/17/07).

[6] Foster is quoting from F. L. Dunn, "Traditional; Asian Medicine and Cosmopolitan Medicine as Adaptive Systems," in C. Leslie (ed.), *Asian Medical Systems* (Berkeley: University of California Press, 1976), p. 135.

[7] Sick people are treated differently than those who are well. They are temporarily released from their responsibilities (e.g., school, work) and are taken care of by others, but they are also expected to work toward getting well.

[8] Some diseases, especially syndromes like AIDS, Lyme disease, and Posttraumatic Stress Disorder, however, can manifest differently. AIDS, for example, presents differently in men and women, and individual bodies often have unique reactions to pharmaceuticals.

Chapter 2

Historical Origins of
Medical Systems

Traditional medical systems are embedded in the cultures in
which they develop and are a product of the local context in which
human beings live their lives. This chapter provides the historical context for the development of medical systems from the Upper Paleolithic
(42,000–12,000 years ago) to the present (see Table 2.1).[1] We begin with
a discussion of the ways that human behavior and subsistence strategies have shaped the patterns of morbidity and mortality to which prehistoric healers and those that have followed them have had to
respond. We then turn to the historically documented medical traditions from the early civilizations of Mesopotamia, Egypt, India, and
China. These traditions preceded those of Greece, Rome, and Persia,
which were the precursors of medieval and modern European medicine. The medical texts from Greece and Rome were protected and augmented by Persian physicians and scholars after the fall of the Greek
and Roman empires. At the end of the Persian state era, the texts were
preserved in Europe by the Catholic Church during the Middle Ages, a
time when professional medicine receded and monks, nuns, and folk
healers dominated the healing arts in the Western world. During the
Renaissance, these ancient medical texts and healing practices from
the early Western civilizations provided the base for the development
of modern medicine in Europe, which ultimately evolved into Western
biomedicine after the scientific revolution and the extraordinary
advances in biology (e.g., discovery of the circulation of the blood, anesthesia, vaccines) and pharmacology (e.g., antibiotics, antiviral drugs,

Table 2.1   Events Associated with the Emergence of the Great Medical Systems.

Era or Civilization	Year*	Events
Upper Paleolithic	40,000–10,000 BCE	Emergence of regionally distinctive cultures
Agricultural Origins	20,000–10,000 BCE	Beginnings of agriculture
Mesopotamia Sumeria Babylonia Phoenicia	3100–1600 BCE 3100–2000 BCE 2000–1600 BCE 950–146 BCE	Clay tablets, cuneiform script Interactions with Greece and Rome
Egypt	3000 BCE–500 CE	Papyri with medical texts
India	4500–2000 BCE 1000–800 BCE ca. 500 BCE	Vedas Ayurvedic texts Persian and Greek invasions
China	3000 ± 300 BCE 2000 BCE 1800–1300 BCE 300 BCE	I Ching Yin/yang principle established First writings, oracle bones Yellow Emperor's 18 volume classic
Greece	460–361 BCE 479–449 BCE 427–347 BCE 356–323 BCE ca. 323–30 BCE	Hippocrates (4 humors & balance) Persian wars Plato and Aristotle Alexander the Great Hellenistic period
Roman Empire	14 BCE–37 CE 40–80 130–200 324–395 330	*On Medicine*, Celsus *De Materia Medica*, Dioscorides Galen Christian Roman Empire (West) Byzantine Empire established (East)
Persian State	560 BCE–636 CE 570–632 850–923 980–1037 1200–1400	Muhammad's prophetic medicine Al-Razi (Rhazes) Ibn Sina (Avicenna) Mongol invasions
Middle Ages Europe	500–1500	Disease as test of faith, Catholic Church
Europe and North America	1300–1650 1450–1630 1578–1657 1750–1830 1840 1822–1895 1940–1950 2003	Renaissance Scientific Revolution Harvey (circulation of blood) Industrialization Surgical anesthesia Louis Pasteur (vaccines) Antibiotics Human genome map completed

* BCE: before Christian era; CE: current era

14

chemotherapy) that followed it, finally culminating with current advances in immunology, neurology, and the mapping of the human genome. We shall see clearly in this chapter that, like the current globalization of access to medical systems, there has been an enormous, albeit somewhat slower paced, amount of contact among various cultures, societies, civilizations, and empires and their medical systems for most of recorded history.

MEDICAL SYSTEMS AND SUBSISTENCE STRATEGIES

*[handwritten margin note: * Our social organization is embodied in our biology (mediates our interaction with the environment, etc)]*

The broad patterns of morbidity *(disease)* and mortality *(death)* among human beings stem from our own biology, our interaction with local environments (e.g., resource extraction, local flora and fauna, weather, terrain, etc.), the ways we have made our living (i.e., subsistence and production strategies), and the social systems and structures that have defined human social relationships. Healing systems have to respond to the primary immediate causes of morbidity in the societies in which they develop. These disease patterns are shaped by ways in which people use their environment and the kind of social organization they have developed. There are five general types of human subsistence strategies traditionally recognized in anthropology that broadly describe the range of human subsistence and technological patterns: (1) hunting, gathering, and foraging, (2) horticulture, (3) nomadic herding, (4) peasant agriculture, and (5) industrial (Janzen 2002, McElroy and Townsend 2004). To these, we add global modernity and the information society (Janes 1999) characteristic of our globalized planet today. Each of these subsistence strategies is characterized by specific kinds of ecological interaction and morbidity and mortality patterns (see Table 2.2). They are not mutually exclusive strategies, and no hierarchy of increasing modernity is intended in this discussion. Rather, in different parts of the world at most points in time with the exception of our earliest existence as hunters and foragers, two or more of these strategies have coexisted as they still do today. The important point is that different subsistence strategies result in different disease patterns that must be understood in order to understand the development of healing systems.

The Upper Paleolithic Era

The first civilizations in the old world developed around 3500 to 1500 BCE and the oldest written medical traditions date from this time in Mesopotamia, Egypt, India, and China. Before that we have information about human disease, diet, and certain kinds of healing practices

Table 2.2   Disease Patterns and Subsistence Strategies

	Population/Fertility	Subsistence	Diet	Morbidity & Mortality Pattern	Types of Healing Practitioners
Hunter-Gatherers	Slow growth Mean about 3 children Life expectancy at birth about 30 yrs Small family groups	Nomadic Hunting & fishing Gathering	Seasonal shortages Varied Good	Endemic diseases Parasitic diseases Injuries/Accidents Interpersonal violence Warfare Old age	Shaman Healer
Horticulturalists	Slow growth Mean about 3 children Life expectancy at birth about 35 yrs Small–medium, usually kin-based groups	Seminomadic Gardening Gathering Hunting & fishing Some domestic animals	Protein shortages Protein/calorie ratio Less varied Generally good Reliance on tubers	Endemic diseased Parasitic diseases Epidemic diseases Dietary deficiencies (especially children) Injuries/Accidents Interpersonal violence Warfare Old age	Shaman Healer
Nomadic Herders	Slow growth Life expectancy unknown Small–medium, usually kin-based groups—little known	Seminomadic Herd animals Gardening Trade with agricultural villages	Little known Meat & milk Little known	Endemic diseases Parasitic diseases Injuries/Accidents Interpersonal violence Warfare Old age	Shaman Healer
Peasant Agriculturalists	High growth Mean about 5–6 children Shorter birth intervals—2 years Life expectancy at birth about 35–45 years Towns, villages, first cities/civilizations	Sedentary Farming & gardening Domestic animals Hunting & fishing Gathering	Protein, calorie, vitamin & mineral shortages Crop failures Rice, wheat, corn, millet & sorghum Generally good Seasonal shortages	Endemic diseases Parasitic diseases Epidemic diseases Dietary deficiencies (especially children) Injuries/Accidents Interpersonal violence Warfare Old age	Shaman Healer Midwife Medium Priest Witch/sorcerer Physicians Surgeons

	Population/ Fertility	Subsistence	Diet	Morbidity & Mortality Pattern	Types of Healing Practitioners
Developed (North, First World)	Slow or negative growth *Mean 1.6 children *Life expectancy at birth = 77 years Large populations, cities, towns, villages	Mixed sedentary & migration	Overnutrition Cash-based shortages	Chronic diseases Lifestyle/behavioral Psycho-social Industrial/technology related Injuries Accidents Interpersonal violence Warfare Old age HIV/AIDS	Shaman Healer Midwife Medium Priest Witch/sorcerer Physicians Allied health professionals Public health
		Market economy	Highly varied High meat, fat Processed foods		
Less-Developed (South, Third World)	High growth transitioning to slower growth *Mean 2.9 children (3.4 when excluding China) *Life expectancy at birth = 66 years (63 when excluding China) Large populations, mega cities, towns, villages	Seasonal labor migration Mixed sedentary & migration	Protein, calorie, vitamin & mineral shortages Cash-based shortages Crop shortages	Endemic diseases Parasitic diseases Epidemic diseases Dietary deficiencies Chronic diseases Lifestyle/behavioral Psycho-social Industrial/technology related Injuries/Accidents Interpersonal violence Warfare Old age HIV/AIDS	Shaman Healer Midwife Medium Priest Witch/sorcerer Physicians Allied health professionals Public health
		Market economy Farming Cash cropping Subsistence Gardening	Varied Processed foods		

*Population Reference Bureau, World Population Data Sheet 2006.

from the Upper Paleolithic Era (40,000–10,000 BCE) when our ancestors lived as hunter-gatherers only from the fossil record, from studies
of human and animal remains (e.g., bones, teeth, and soft tissues preserved in burial practices like mummification or by accident in ashes,
ice, bogs/tar pits, coprolites), and from prehistoric artistic endeavors
(e.g., depictions of recognizable diseases on pottery, masks, paintings).
Paleopathologists who study diseases of the past have documented a
number of infectious diseases (e.g., tuberculosis), chronic conditions
(e.g., osteoarthritis, rheumatoid arthritis, malignant bone tumors),
dietary insufficiency diseases (e.g., rickets, which leaves its mark on
bones), common injuries (e.g., broken bones), inflicted trauma (e.g.,
spear wounds or carnivore bites), congenital defects (e.g., dwarfism),
and dental caries. They have also documented surgical intervention
through trepanation, the removal of a small disk of bone from the skull
(Zimmerman 2004).

Anthropologists have documented the population, subsistence,
dietary, and morbidity and mortality patterns of human beings who
lived as hunter-gatherers both in the present and historically (see
McElroy and Townsend 2004). From such studies we know that hunter-
gatherer groups lived in low population densities, often in small family
groups (see Table 2.2). Life expectancy[2] was much lower than today;
then it was age 28–30 compared to age 65 in less-developed and 77 in
more developed countries today (Population Reference Bureau 2006).
Women had a relatively small number of children—about three to four
births (Boserup 1981:37–38). The hunting and gathering life required
a nomadic or semi-nomadic existence that resulted in a good, varied
diet with seasonal shortages as the main dietary constraint. Threats to
human morbidity and mortality included endemic diseases, parasites,
injuries, accidents, interpersonal violence, and diseases of aging. These
morbidity and mortality patterns are similar to those suggested by the
Paleolithic remains of our ancestors. We infer from studies of hunter-
gatherer groups that most healers in these dispersed groups were probably shamans and herbalists.

The Shift to Agriculture and Early States

The origins of agriculture date from between 11,500 BCE in the
Near East to about 4500 BCE in West Africa; by 2000 BCE, most human
beings in the world were dependent on agriculture (Bodley 2000, Diamond 1999), although in remote areas hunting and gathering societies
survived as well. With the shift to agriculture, new patterns of subsistence emerged among human populations—semi-nomadic horticulture
(tuber-based—e.g., manioc, yams) usually mixed with hunting and
fishing or domestic animal husbandry; nomadic herding (dairy and
meat), probably mixed with gathering and trade for grain crops; and

peasant agriculture based on the major grain crops of the region (i.e., corn, rice, wheat, sorghum, millet) with domestic animal husbandry also varying by region (e.g., chickens, turkeys, ducks, pigs, goats, cows, guinea pigs, and sheep for food, eggs, and milk; dogs, horses, camels, water buffalo, and llamas, mostly as working stock).

The shift to dependence on cultivated food and domestic animals created new patterns of morbidity and mortality for humans that included dietary insufficiency and deficiency diseases (e.g., protein-calorie malnutrition, anemia, pellagra, scurvy) related to seasonal shortages and the kinds of crops grown and diffused animal diseases related to their domestication (e.g., avian flu, cow pox) (Armelagos et al. 1991). Farming allowed higher population densities in settled villages and towns that resulted in the increased importance of infectious diseases and epidemics that are dependent on a large population living in close proximity for transmission (e.g., small pox, measles, plague, flu, malaria) and in diseases related to environmental hygiene, especially those involving fecal-oral and water-borne transmission (e.g., diarrhea, cholera, schistosomiasis).

Although little can be determined about medical systems in cultures with no recorded history, analogy can be made to existing or historically recorded traditional medical systems of groups living under similar conditions. Most anthropologists and historians infer from studies of ethnohistorical and contemporary ethnomedical systems among recent or contemporary hunter-gatherer, horticultural, nomadic, and peasant farmer groups that prehistoric paleomedical and post-agricultural healing techniques probably consisted of both empirical and magical or spiritual techniques. Empirical techniques include remedies ingested or applied that use local plant, animal, and mineral substances in their preparation (e.g., herbal remedies, spider webs to stop bleeding), bone setting, and midwifery—all of which were learned from observation, practice, experimentation, and oral transmission and were rooted in an extensive empirical knowledge of the natural world. Magical or spiritual techniques address disease and other misfortunes (e.g., mental illness, miscarriage, droughts, insect plagues) that are believed by adherents to be caused by supernatural forces or beings. Magico-spiritual healers include priests, shamans, witches, diviners, and lesser healers (e.g., diagnosticians, spirit mediums) specialized in mediating between humans and supernatural forces to restore harmony between them and thus eliminate illness (Foster and Anderson 1978, Magner 2005, McElroy and Townsend 2004, Scrimshaw 2001).

Early Civilizations: Mesopotamia and Egypt

With the development of the first civilizations (defined by presence written records), we have the first medical texts with written descriptions of diseases and their treatments and the emergence of physicians as a professional class of healers (Tables 2.1 and 2.2). Some of the cuneiform stone tablets from the Sumerian civilization (3100–2000 BCE) in Mesopotamia for example, included both medical (e.g., symptoms and therapies to remedy them) and magical (e.g., omens for divining cause and prognosis) information related to illness and healing and suggest that the common health problems of Sumerians included schistosomiasis (a parasitic worm), dysentery, pneumonia, epilepsy, eye disorders, and malnutrition (Magner 2005). By the Babylonian era (2000–1600 BCE), there were laws pertaining to surgeons, veterinarians, midwives, and wet nurses, recorded in the *Code of Hammurabi* (ca. 1700 BCE), suggesting that specialization in healing roles existed at that time. The first named physician in history, Imhotep, practiced at the court of Pharaoh Zoser (ca. 2980 BCE) in ancient Egypt and eventually became a deity in the eyes of his people. The first lengthy medical treatise also dates from this area (the Ebers papyrus, ca. 1500 BCE). Thus, evidence from both Mesopotamia and Egypt suggests that early on (3000–1700 BCE) specialization and professionalization in the medical arts had evolved (Magner 2005). By the time of the Phoenician civilization (950–146 BCE), there was much interaction, both peaceful and hostile, among the peoples of the circum-Mediterranean area, and a sharing of medical knowledge across cultures, a pattern that has continued ever since.

In Egypt (3000 BCE–500 CE), medicine was inextricably tied to religion. Each part of the body was ruled by its own god. There were specialized physicians for the eyes, head, teeth, and stomach, suggesting that ailments of these organs were particularly common. Egyptian medical theory posited that while humans were born healthy, the body was innately susceptible to diseases caused by intestinal putrefaction, external entities (winds, worms, ghosts and spirits), and overly strong emotions. Healing required ridding the body of disease-causing entities through purging or exorcism. The Ebers papyrus lists prescriptions (700 drugs and 800 formulas), diseases and surgeries, and incantations and may have been a reference for physicians, surgeons, and exorcists. Studies of mummies have determined that disease burdens in ancient Egypt included parasitic worms (including schistosomiasis), pneumoconiosis (caused by sand in the lungs), tuberculosis, arthritis, and trauma. Endemic schistosomiasis may have been one of the reasons for the ancient Egyptians' preoccupation with intestinal putrefaction since infection often leads to liver, intestine, or bladder damage. Similarly, the winds referenced in causation theories may well have led to eye problems and infections, which are still a problem in contemporary Egypt, especially trachoma, a leading cause of preventable blindness.

Perhaps the Egyptian concern with intestinal putrefaction combined with their intense interest in life after death was a factor in the funerary practice of mummification, which entailed removing the viscera, except the heart, and drying the body thoroughly with hot sand, embalming it with vinegar brine, or packing it with natron (sodium carbonate, a natural desiccant), a process that could take up to 70 days, after which it was wrapped in linen and placed in a wooden case. Such practices might ensure eternal rest free from the ravages of intestinal disorders. Although those who prepared the body this way had first-hand knowledge of the internal organs, this knowledge was apparently not used in medical treatment. In fact, except for the treatment of injuries, both accidental and battle related, there was virtually no systematic study of the anatomy and physiology of the human body, except for a brief period in Alexandria during the Hellenistic period (ca. 323–30 BCE), until the Renaissance in Europe when artists and anatomists reformed the field (Magner 2005).

THE GREAT HISTORICAL MEDICAL TRADITIONS

In contrast to the incomplete information available for ancient Egypt and Mesopotamia, there are three great classical medical traditions[3] that have extensive, written documentation from India, China, and Greece. These healing systems respectively are Ayurvedic medicine, Traditional Chinese medicine (TCM), and Greek medicine. Ayurvedic medicine and TCM persist to this day as distinct medical traditions, while Greek medicine survives in the theory and practice of contemporary Unani medicine in Asia and the Middle East. Greek medicine gave rise to the European medical traditions that developed after the scientific revolution into modern biomedicine.

Ayurvedic Medicine

Roughly contemporary to the medical developments in Egypt and Mesopotamia, was the independent development of the great medical traditions in India (4500–500 BCE) and China (2000–300 BCE). The oldest references to medical practice in India date to the Vedas, sacred Hindu texts, and include legends about gods and healers intervening with disease-causing demons to restore health and well-being, diverse medical lore, descriptions of internal anatomy, accounts of wounds and diseases, mention of over 1,000 healing herbs, and the text of spells (Magner 2005, Lad 1995). Illness was thought to be the result of sin or the work of demons. Healers—magicians, surgeons, and physicians—used confession, exorcism, charms, incantations, and herbal remedies as cure and prevention.

The basic Ayurvedic medical texts date from 1000 to 800 BCE (Magner 2005). Ayurveda is known as the science of life. Its objective was the prevention of disease and the maintenance of health rather than the treatment of disease. Health was secured by maintaining balance in the three *doshas*, or humors (wind, bile, and phlegm or, alternately, motion, energy, and inertia), which when combined with blood determined the vital functions of the body (see Table 2.3). Health also depended on sustaining harmony between the humors and body tissues; normal digestion and elimination; and gratification of the senses, the mind, and the soul. The body was made up of five elements (earth, water, fire, wind, and ether/space) and the seven *dhatu*, or body tissues (blood, muscle, fat, bone, nerves, semen, ova). In addition, there were 107 vital points (*marmas*) in the body that were individually named and referred to specific places where injuries were likely to be serious or fatal (Kurup 1983, Lad 1995, Magner 2005).

Deficiencies or excesses of one or more humors predisposed the body to certain kinds of illnesses by causing disturbances in the blood. Balance could be restored through proper diet and behavior, exercise, fasting, purging, blood letting, herbal remedies and other Ayurvedic medicines, and surgery (Magner 2005). Diagnosis was made by careful attention to the patient's narrative and the physician's physical assessment (e.g., appearance, pulse, tongue, urine, listening to the heart and lungs) (Kurup 1983). Surgery, important in all times and places with respect to warfare, was particularly well developed in ancient India as was the art of plastic surgery for reconstructing the nose, lips, and ears (Magner 2005).

Other traditions affecting Ayurvedic medical beliefs included the quasi-medical ideas embedded in religious ideas about karma, the life cycle, yoga, diet, exercise, hygiene, meditation, and astrology (Lad 1995, Magner 2005). The idea of a life force or vital energy (*shakti,* in Hindiusm the personification of God's female aspect) that animated the body, while a more central aspect of Traditional Chinese medicine, made its way into Indian healing by way of ideas about male (*purusha*) and female (*prakruti*) energy, yoga, and meditation techniques to raise cosmic consciousness (Lad 1995). All of these philosophies deal with the place of the individual in the universe and in relation to other people, to the spiritual world, and to the environment, and the necessity of maintaining harmony in the body and in social and spiritual relationships. The practice of moderation in living, compassion for others, and respect for the gods/spirits was important for a long and healthy life.

Today, Ayurvedic medicine is an officially recognized medical system (as is biomedicine) in much of West and Southeast Asia, where it is an important source of medical care, especially in Bangladesh, India, Nepal, Pakistan, and Sri Lanka, and wherever migrants from those areas have settled (e.g., the Americas, Europe, Africa, Southeast Asia) (Bannerman et al. 1983).

Traditional Chinese Medicine

Traditional Chinese medicine (TCM) also has a long history although the Vedas predate the first Chinese writings by almost 2,000 years. While much of the historical development of TCM is couched in myth, the basic foundation can be found in the *I Ching* (The Book of Changes) that outlines the Chinese philosophy of dynamic balance of opposites and the acceptance of the inevitability of change. There are no firm dates for the origin of *I Ching*, but scholars believe it was written about 3000 ± 300 BCE. The 18-volume classic, *Nei Ching* (The Yellow Emperor's Classic of Internal Medicine), dates from 300 BCE and sets forth the principles that have guided TCM for 2,500 years—the balance of yin and yang, the five phases or elements and the correlations among them, and the factors that impinge on human life (e.g., family, food, environment). Chinese medicine is guided by the idea that the world is a single, unbroken wholeness (*Tao*) that exists within every person, each of whom is a microcosm of the universe. TCM is embedded in nature, couched in naturalistic symbols and metaphors, and "living processes are seen as a mosaic of connected relationships and conditions . . . the human body is viewed as an ecosystem, and the language of . . . medicine is based on metaphors from nature" (Beinfield and Korngold 1995:45).

Yin and yang (e.g., earth/heaven, cold/heat, shadow/sun, female/male) are polar opposites that cannot exist without each other and whose dynamic balance/imbalance can cause illness. Yin and yang are the basis of life. They give rise to the five phases/elements: earth, metal, water, wood, and fire, which, in turn are linked to each other by relationships of generation and destruction,[4] a part of the larger idea of continual change on which the basic philosophy of TCM rests. The body is comprised of qi[5] (an animating force or energy), moisture (body fluids), and blood (body tissues). The basic body organs, five firm yin organs (heart, spleen, lungs, liver, kidneys) and five hollow yang organs (gall bladder, bladder, stomach, large intestines, small intestines), are related to the five phases/elements. They are linked by a system of conduits within the body through which qi flows. In TCM, anatomy is thought of in terms of function rather than structure (as in biomedicine). For example, an organ called the triple warmer, which has no anatomical reality, is an important part of Chinese functional anatomy. It is an energy system that manages the digestive process through the flow of fluids in digestion, transportation, and excretion (Magner 2005).

In TCM, health is achieved through maintaining a balance of all the contending forces (yin/yang, phases/elements) and a free flow of qi. Illness results from a blockage or depletion of qi or an imbalance of yin and yang or the phases/elements. Diagnostic techniques include patient narratives and physical assessment by the physician (e.g., appearance, 50 pulses, tongue, temperature, joint flexibility, sensitivity of 365 acupuncture points, moisture of skin), which are directed towards determining the prevailing balance in the body. Preventive measures include a moderate lifestyle and attention to the careful balancing of hot/cold and moist/dry in daily living. Treatment attempts to restore balance by use of acupuncture to readjust the qi, moxibustion (a combination of acupuncture and burning of mugwort, a medicinal plant), medicines (animal, mineral, and vegetable—including use of over 5,000 herbs), diet, and exercise.

It has been estimated that over one-third of humanity has relied on TCM for care. Today, TCM is one of the official medical systems in China. It flourishes alongside biomedicine.

Greek and Roman Medicine

The third of the great medical traditions came from ancient Greece where the foundations for Western philosophy, science, and medicine originated. Although historians believe that Greek medicine was well developed by the time Homer set down the oral traditions of the *Iliad* and the *Odyssey* in the 8th century BCE, it is Hippocrates (460–361 BCE), who is remembered as the "Father of Medicine," and his words "At least do no harm" have descended through the ages as the most well known part of the *Hippocratic Oath*, still taken by graduates of some medical schools (Magner 2005). The basic underlying principle of Hippocratic medicine is that nature is a strong healing force and the duty of the physician is to help the body to restore balance and heal itself. Hippocrates was, perhaps, the first to explain disease as a natural process that could be understood through rational study rather than the result of supernatural agents. He also suggested that health and disease could be affected by the physical environment and by social, religious, and political institutions. To treat the patient, the physician had to understand his/her temperament and pay attention to how disease was related to the patient's way of living, especially food and drink, and application of the principle of humoral medicine (hot/cold balance or opposition) in curing. In addition, astrology[6] played a role in Greek notions of the body in that physical type was thought to be associated with zodiac and planetary alignments at the time of birth. Astrology was used to predict auspicious and inauspicious times for events, the relationships between healing plants and heavenly bodies, and prediction of the course of illness based on the time the person fell ill (Ackernecht 1982, Magner 2005).

In Greek medicine, the ultimate cause of disease was seen as an imbalance in the four humors (yellow bile, blood, phlegm, and black bile), which were associated with four elements (fire, air, water, and earth) and four states (hot, cold, moist, dry). Health was a balanced blending of the humors. A person's temperament, or personality type, was associated with how much of each humor was present in his/her body. The choleric, hot tempered, temperament was associated with an abundance of yellow bile, with the element fire, and with the hot-dry state; the sanguine, sturdy and cheerful temperament with an abundance of blood, the element air, and the hot-moist state; the phlegmatic, slow and dull, temperament with an abundance of phlegm, the element water, and the moist-cold state; and finally the melancholy, sad, depressed temperament with an abundance of black bile, the element earth, and the cold-dry state. Humoral theory was used to restore a balance among the humors and to assist the body's natural healing forces. By rationalizing disease, Hippocrates attacked the ignorance and superstition surrounding many diseases previously thought to be supernatural punishments (e.g., epilepsy) and treated them all as natural processes. Hippocrates, 12 centuries ago, presaged biomedical understanding that diseases—both individual (e.g., leprosy) and epidemic (e.g., HIV/AIDS)—are natural processes, not supernatural punishment. He also recognized the social and political impact on health (Magner 2005).

The Greek physicians used the standard techniques of diagnosis observation, patient narrative, taking the pulse, and examining the urine. They were also adept at treating wounds, fractures, and other injuries through surgery. They used a wide array of medicines made from animal, mineral, and vegetable products and also cupping, venesection, and scarification. Greek medicine, like the other great medical traditions, however, was powerless against the infectious diseases that ravaged the old world especially plague and malaria, which are thought to have contributed significantly to the decline of the Greek civilization.

Greco-Roman and Greco-Islamic Medicine

Alexander the Great (356–323 BCE) conquered much of what was known of the old world (the eastern circum-Mediterranean area and parts of western Asia) after inheriting a unified Greece from his father. Alexander's empire included the Persian Empire, Anatolia (now Turkey), Syria, Phoenicia, Gaza, Egypt, Bactria (now Afghanistan), and Macedonia, extending his empire to the Punjab in northern India. Alexandria, a city northwest of the Nile River delta, was founded by and named for Alexander. It became a prominent cultural, political, and economic metropolis and was the site of a great library and museum where Greek medical and other intellectual traditions flourished, and where human dissection was, perhaps for the first time, a regular part of medical learning (Magner 2005).

Unfortunately, most of the texts in the library in Alexandria were lost over the next 250 years. The first assault on the library occurred during riots that ensued after Julius Caesar arrived (48 BCE) and extended the Roman Empire to Egypt. Later, Christian leaders were responsible for the destruction of many of the pagan reminders of Alexandria's past. By 395, there were no more scientists and philosophers left in Alexandria, and the Persian conquest (642–646) resulted in the final destruction of the library. Nevertheless, for some 200 years the library and museum complex at Alexandria was a center of learning for scholars from all parts of the known world, and much sharing of ideas about medicine and the healing arts must have occurred there (Magner 2005).

Greek medicine persisted as the dominant medical system of the Roman Empire, and most of the physicians used by the Romans were Greek. The first Western book on the use of herbs in healing, *De Materia Medica*, was written by a Greek physician named Dioscorides (ca. 40–80), who outlined various herbal remedies and the characteristics of the plants used to make them. Earlier, a Roman scholar, Celsus (ca. 14 BCE–37 CE), divided medical curing into three types: diet and lifestyle, medication, and surgery in his account of Roman medical traditions called *On Medicine* (Magner 2005).

Even though Hippocrates is the father of modern medicine, it was Galen (130–200) who proposed the idea that therapy had to be based in an understanding of the anatomy and physiology of the human body and who, thus, laid the foundation for modern scientific medicine. Galen also rejected the application of astrology to medicine, although he maintained that astrology was important to understanding life and nature in general. Galen's ideas dominated Western medical thought in Europe until the 16th century. His writings were also the major medical resources for the Persian physician-scholars, Al-Razi (Rhazes, 850–923) and Ibn Sina (Avicenna, 980–1037), whose own writings preserved the Greek medical traditions during the European Middle Ages and contributed to the Arab adaptation of secular Greek medicine, called Unani (Unan is Arabic for Greece) (Magner 2005).

The other major medical tradition in Persia was the religious medical tradition known as Prophetic medicine coupled with the Islamic teaching that faith was the way to deal with illness. Prophetic medicine advocated traditional medical practices current during the Prophet Muhammad's lifetime (570–632) and also those mentioned in the Qur'an rather than those assimilated from Hellenistic society. Therapy (prevention and treatment) consisted of diet, medicines (e.g., honey), bloodletting, and cautery, but unlike Greek medicine, did not include surgery. After the fall of the Roman Empire, these Greco-Roman medical traditions survived in the centers of learning in Persia (500–1500) and in Moorish Spain (711–1492). Today, the Unani medical tradition is an important source of medical care mainly in India and Pakistan (Bannerman et al. 1983, Brewer 2004, Magner 2005).

COMPARISON OF THE
GREAT MEDICAL TRADITIONS

These three great medical traditions—Ayurvedic, Chinese, Greek—clearly share core elements in their respective theories of disease causation, prevention, and treatment; although each has its own idiosyncratic features (see Table 2.3). Certainly, the idea of (im)balance is a key organizing component for understanding health in all three healing traditions. So, too, is the importance placed on humors and elements as vital components of the body that must be in harmony to maintain health. In all three medical systems, imbalance causes illness, and restoration of balance through diet, lifestyle, and use of medicines or surgery is necessary to restore health.

Chinese medicine differs from the other two traditions in that the philosophy of qi, the vital life force, replaces that of the humors. The free flow of qi and its blockage or imbalance are causes of health and illness, respectively. Tai Chi, an ancient system of exercise and movement techniques, is designed to maintain the balance of qi. Acupuncture, too, is unique to Chinese medicine and is used to realign the flow of qi in the body. It is likely that Chinese medicine was more isolated from the other two traditions during its early development, both because of its geographical location and the historical tendency of the Chinese toward isolationism, largely motivated by external threat. However, with the opening of the Silk Road[7] in the 2nd century BCE, there was much more contact between China and Central Asia and through it with the Western world. In fact, Buddhism and later Islam as well as trade goods came to China along the Silk Road.

It is most interesting that diagnosis in these three prescientific medical traditions predate the use of what are now the signature diagnostic techniques of biomedicine—observation of the patient's overall physical and emotional presentation, the patient's verbal history, palpation, pulse taking, and examination of bodily fluids and function. Similarly, prevention hinges on maintaining a moderate lifestyle and avoidance of behaviors and things known to make one ill, themes that are the hallmarks of preventive medicine today.

Finally, although most fully developed in Greek medicine, the idea that hot/cold and moist/dry properties of humors, diseases, food, and medicine influence health and illness is an underlying principle regarding health maintenance in all three systems. There are also magical elements in each of the three systems seen most notably in ideas about the influence of astrology on a person's temperament and life events.

Table 2.3. Basic Principles of the Great Classical Medical Traditions.

	Indian/ Ayurvedic	Chinese/TCM	Greek/Greek Medicine	Unani/Arab Adaptation of Greek Medicine
Humors	3 doshas wind/motion bile/energy phlegm/inertia	Yin/yang	4 humors blood phlegm yellow bile black bile	4 humors blood phlegm yellow bile black bile
Life Force Energy	Shakti	Qi (Chi)		
Elements	5 elements fire earth water air/wind ether	5 elements fire earth water metal wood	4 elements fire (heat) earth (dry) water (moist) air (cold)	4 elements fire (heat) earth (dry) water (moist) air (cold)
Composition of the body	Blood, muscle, fat, bone, nerves, semen, ova	Channel system Meridians	4 humors 4 elements	4 humors 4 elements
Cause of disease	Imbalance of doshas Temperament	Imbalance of elements or yin/yang Blocked Qi	Nature Imbalance of humors Temperament	Nature Imbalance of humors Temperament
Diagnosis	Observation Patient report Pulse Tongue Urine	Observation Patient report Pulse Tongue	Observation Patient report Pulse Urine	Observation Patient report Pulse Urine
Prevention	Moderate lifestyle Yoga Energy flow Vegetarianism	Tea Acupuncture Energy flow Wine/fruit	Moderate lifestyle Diet Wine Honey	Moderate lifestyle Diet Honey
Treatment	Medicines Fasting/purging Bloodletting Diet/exercise Surgery	Medicines Acupuncture Moxibustion Diet/exercise	Medicines Bloodletting Cupping Diet/exercise Surgery	Medicines Bloodletting Cupping Diet/exercise
Hot/cold	Food	Food Yin/yang	Food Disease Medications Humors	Food Disease Medications Humors
Other	Temperament Astrology Zodiac	Astrology Numerology	Temperament Astrology	Temperament

These three great medical traditions have affected local ethno-medical systems in the areas in which they developed and their influence has spread well beyond their geographic origins through migration, exploration, religious proselytizing, trade, war, imperialism, colonialism, and deliberate study and borrowing. In their present day versions, Traditional Chinese, Ayurvedic, and Unani medicine continue to influence each other and also biomedicine and the many complementary and alternative medicines and traditional therapies in existence around the globe.

European Middle Ages

During the Middle Ages in Europe after the fall of the Roman Empire, all secular learning became inferior to the theological explanations of the Christian Church. The spirit of inquiry that had led to the developments in Greco-Roman medicine and other sciences was the opposite of what was demanded of Christians—faith in God and adherence to the teachings of the Church. In medieval Christianity, disease was thought to be a test of faith or a punishment from God, who alone could heal. Suffering was a natural condition of mankind that could only be alleviated through faith in God. This religious philosophy of illness and curing, like that of Islamic Prophetic medicine, was at odds with the naturalistic philosophy that had guided Greco-Roman medicine until this time. Although secular healing practices continued to exist alongside religious healing as they do today, the meaning of illness was interpreted quite differently. The therapeutic arsenal of secular medicine—diet, drugs, bleeding, and surgery—treated bodily ills. Religious medicine, by contrast, used prayer, incantations, penitence, exorcism, holy relics, and charms to alleviate illness and suffering (Magner 2005).

Miraculous healing became a dominant theme during the Middle Ages, especially through petition to saints or contact with their relics. Some saints became associated with the healing of particular diseases or disorders. However, by the 9th century, the study of medicine had been reincorporated into Christian studies, and by the 12th century, there were faculties of medicine in European universities that were mostly associated with monasteries that had libraries, herbal gardens, hospitals, and infirmaries on their grounds. Kings and other nobles had court physicians and surgeons to treat those wounded in battle. As medicine developed into a profession, laws were enacted to control its practice and that of other types of healing practitioners (e.g., surgeons, midwives, bone setters, veterinarians, tooth extractors, etc.) (Magner 2005). Until the 20th century, surgery and medicine were two separate healing traditions. Physicians practiced internal medicine. Surgeons belonged to the same guild as barbers, and success in surgery depended on speed and physical strength. Only after the development of the means to control infection and pain (antibiotics and analgesics) in the latter 19th century, which improved patient survival rates, did surgery come to enjoy the power and prestige that it has today. Before that, it was much despised as a manual trade. With these scientific developments, however, by 1900, surgery was accepted within the field of medicine and moved into the hospitals (Starr 1982).

Medieval Spain had quite a different history from the rest of Europe. In 711, North African Muslims (Moors) attacked Gibraltar and took the Iberian Peninsula in three years, dominating Spain for 700 years until King Ferdinand and Queen Isabella completed the Christian *Reconquista* (reconquest) of Spain in 1492, routing the last Moorish stronghold from Granada in the same year that Columbus stumbled upon the New World and ushered in Spain's Golden Age (1500–1600) of exploration and domination of the Americas. The Moorish culture in Spain was arguably Europe's most advanced and tolerant center of learning during the Middle Ages (especially 800–1000), preserving Greek and Arabic texts on mathematics, astronomy, medicine, and other subjects in the great libraries of Córdoba where translations into Latin were undertaken (Menocal 2002).

Beginning with the Renaissance (1300) and into the modern era there was increasing written documentation of the theoretical and philosophical principles underlying healing systems in Europe that culminated in the development of biomedicine in the West. As the seafaring states of Europe began exploring and colonizing the globe, they brought with them not only Christianity but also their medical system, which was, in the 1500s, still based largely on Greek medical principles. Hence, early on, ideas about bodily humors and hot/cold balance were spread by Spanish conquistadors, priests, and settlers throughout the New World and to colonies in Asia where they were incorporated into or existed alongside local indigenous medical beliefs. Indigenous medical systems also enriched (figuratively and monetarily) Western systems with the introduction of herbs and medicines from the colonies (e.g., *cinchona* and tobacco from the Americas and opium from Asia). With the continuing expansion of the European empires abroad during the 1600–1800s, the rapid advances in scientific medicine in the 18th and 19th centuries were also exported worldwide along with the dubious benefits of industrialization. Indeed, many of the advances in infectious disease control were spurred by the need to keep the colonizers healthy in tropical climates (e.g., yellow fever and malaria control during the building of the Panama Canal; the establishment of the London School of Tropical Medicine).[8]

Industrial Societies and Global Modernity

With the industrial revolution (1750–1830), human subsistence patterns changed again. After about 30,000 years as hunter-gatherers and another 14,000 as agriculturalists, it is only the last 250 years that have seen the rise of industrial states with their new health risks and benefits. During most of our human history as hunter-gatherers, horticulturalists, herders, and early agriculturalists, life expectancy was low (about 28–33 years) and population growth was slow (Boserup 1981). The major causes of morbidity and mortality were accidents, injuries, violence, and endemic diseases (Janzen 2002, McElroy and Townsend 2004). The post–agricultural transition improved life expectancy somewhat to 35–55 years but added infectious diseases as a cause of morbidity (Roberts and Manchester 2005). Infectious disease has taken a huge toll on human populations. The great plague known as the Black Death in the Middle Ages (1348–1350) killed an estimated one quarter of the population of Europe, and the influenza pandemic of 1918–1919 was probably the worst epidemic the world has known, killing between 20 and 40 million people worldwide (McElroy and Townsend 2004, McNeill 1976).

After industrialization and better control of infectious diseases through public health measures, life expectancy rose and population growth increased at a rapid rate as mortality among infants and children decreased. This "population explosion" (Ehrlich and Ehrlich 1991) finally seems to have abated, and the current trend is toward slow population growth in much of the developing world and negative growth in the formerly most industrialized, now postindustrial areas of the globe—North America, Europe, Japan, Australia, and New Zealand—and in China, which instituted a strict population control policy in 1979 (see Table 2.2).

Demographic Transition

The demographic transition (Notestein 1945) spawned the epidemiological transition (Omran 1971) in which the major causes of morbidity and mortality worldwide have shifted in the last three decades from infectious diseases (e.g., measles, smallpox, malaria) to chronic conditions (e.g., diabetes, heart disease, cancer), lifestyle- and behavioral-related problems (e.g., alcohol, tobacco, and other drug-related health problems), technology-related accidents and injuries (e.g., transportation and manufacturing accidents), and psychosocial problems (e.g., unipolar major depression, post traumatic stress disorders). More recently, a new set of infectious diseases like HIV/AIDS and a resurgence of old ones like tuberculosis have reminded us that we are not free of infectious disease (Frenk et al. 1993, Hyder and Morrow 2001, Murray and Lopez 1996).

Health Transition

The term health transition is used to describe the combined effects of the demographic and epidemiologic transitions. The health transition model deliberately calls attention to the social, economic, and political factors that affect health. The economic development strategies of third-world countries, for example, have affected health both directly and indirectly. The most dramatic change, perhaps, has been the shift from subsistence to market agricultural economies, which has had profound negative effects on diet and nutrition, migration, urbanization, and poverty and has undermined traditional kin-based social structures. Further exacerbating health and development in the developing countries is the massive debt crisis incurred by countries that borrowed money at low but variable interest rates from the World Bank and the International Monetary Fund (IMF) in the 1960s and 1970s to spur economic development. When interest rates skyrocketed in the 1980s, most countries were not able to pay back their loans, which led many countries to default.[9] This led the World Bank and the IMF to impose structural adjustment policies (SAPs) on debtor countries that promoted privatization and free market economies.[10] Some debtor countries, especially those in Latin America, dollarized[11] their currency in an attempt to keep inflation in check. In most countries, SAPs have had a disastrous effect on health and development as nations were forced to cut back on social spending. This has bred political chaos in some countries, particularly in Africa, where both governments and economies have failed, leading to conflict, famine, and misery (Caldwell et al. 1990, Janes 1999).

Syndemics

Taking the health transition model even further, a syndemic theoretical approach (Singer 1996, Singer and Clair 2003) takes into consideration the interactions among two or more pathogens or disease processes, other health-damaging conditions (e.g., stress, poor nutrition), harmful behavioral complexes (e.g., drug abuse, intimate partner violence), and the social conditions of disease sufferers as critical to understanding the spread of disease, its expression, and health impact at the individual and population levels (Singer et al. 2006). It is important to note that both individual diseases and syndemic patterns are compounded by the gross social and economic inequities that exist throughout the world, including within the wealthiest nations, the effects of which have come to be called health disparities, the excess morbidity and mortality suffered by the economically and socially marginalized.[12] More recently, Singer (2007) introduced the term *ecosyndemics* to refer to the impact of global warming on the spread of diseases to new areas and their contact and potential synergistic interaction with other diseases in those areas. Because of global warming, vector borne diseases, such as malaria and dengue, which are spread by mosquitoes, are being diagnosed in places where they were previously unknown. Singer maintains that ecosyndemics will constitute the plagues of the 21st century. Thus, in global modernity, although patterns of morbidity and mortality have shifted as the global population ages, we have not completely escaped the scourges of our ancestors—infectious disease, accidents, hunger, and violence. Rather, we have only added new ones to the list—chronic disease, technology-related health problems, and now the yet to come impact of global warming.

CONCLUSION

As the European colonies gained their independence in the 18th, 19th, and 20th centuries, scientific medicine continued to exist alongside indigenous medical systems. After World War II, the World Health Organization and other governmental and nongovernmental organizations working to improve health for people living in the less developed countries assured the dominance of biomedicine throughout the world until the recent resurgence of interest in the West with what has come to be called complementary and alternative medicine (CAM). Today, the global pool of medical systems available for patients in search of healing and curing includes Ayurvedic and Unani medicine, Traditional Chinese medicine, biomedicine, CAM, religious-based healing (e.g., Christian, Islamic prophetic, Voodoo), and the myriad local medical systems still in existence throughout the world. It is important to keep in mind that perhaps no local medical system has escaped interaction with one or more of the great historical medical traditions described in this chapter. The history of all medicine(s) is a history of learning, borrowing, and testing different responses to disease and illness, just as the history of cure-seeking at the individual level is the simultaneous, sequential, or circular use of the different sectors of health care (popular, folk, professional) and different medical systems.

In the next chapter we turn to a discussion of the many theories of disease causation that underlie the ethnomedical systems that have been studied by anthropologists, historians, missionaries, and others. Some of these theories strongly echo the disease causation theories of the great medical traditions described in this chapter; others elaborate on more locally produced ideas about what makes people sick.

Notes

[1] By convention, CE won't be used for the current era unless a date range spans BCE–CE.

[2] Life expectancy represents the average life span of a newborn and is an indicator of the overall health of a country. Low life expectancy indicates high infant and child mortality rates or severe conditions (e.g., warfare, famine, epidemics), which bring the average age at death down. Among foragers, people who survive infancy and childhood are likely to live into their 50s or 60s (Hill et al. 2007).

[3] The great medical traditions are designated as such by Western historians of medicine because they have an extensive written canon and have been influential in large parts of the old world for centuries.

[4] The generative/destructive aspects of the elements are illustrated in this way. Earth is a source of metal and when used to make a dam, stops water. Water produces wood and puts out fire. Wood produces fire and wooden plows turn the earth. Metal, when heated, flows like water and can cut wood. Fire produces ash/earth and melts metal.

[5] Qi is sometimes written "ch'i" or "chi" and is pronounced as "chee." It means breath in Mandarin Chinese.

[6] Astrology is magic from a scientific perspective, but still has great hold over many people around the world who believe, at least to some extent, in its ability to determine personality characteristics, disease likelihood, and auspicious timing for important events based on astrological sign (e.g., place, time of birth) and the alignment of the heavenly bodies. It is, perhaps, best understood as a kind of naturalistic determinism of fate and personality that attempts to explain, understand, control, or intervene in the randomness of lived experience.

[7] The Silk Road was a network of caravan and ocean trade routes through Southern Asia that connected today's Xi'an (location of the terra cotta warriors) in China with ancient Antioch (modern Turkey) and Syria on the eastern Mediterranean coast, as well as points farther west. The exchanges among the civilizations along this route were critical for the development of the great civilizations of Ancient Egypt, China, India, and Rome, http://en.wikipedia.org/wiki/Silk_Road (accessed 10/26/05).

[8] The London School of Tropical Medicine founded in 1899 (known as the London School of Tropical Hygiene and Medicine since 1924) was founded at the height of the British Empire to combat the tropical diseases that killed many Europeans in the colonies. So many deaths occurred in West Africa that it was known as the "white man's grave." http://k1.ioe.ac.uk/is/archives/Beginnings/begslshtm1.html (accessed 12/8/05).

[9] "In 1970, the world's poorest countries (roughly 60 countries classified as low-income by the World Bank), owed \$25 billion in debt. . . . By 2002, this was \$523 billion. . . . The developing world now spends \$13 on debt repayment for every \$1 it receives in grants." Anup Shah 2005, http://www.globalissues.org/TradeRelated/Debt/Scale.asp (accessed 9/17/07).

[10] "Structural Adjustment Policies are economic policies which countries must follow in order to qualify for new World Bank and International Monetary Fund (IMF) loans and help them make debt repayments on the older debts owed to commercial banks, governments and the World Bank. . . . SAPs are designed for individual countries but have common guiding principles and features which include export-led growth; privatisation and liberalisation; and the efficiency of the free market." Structural Adjustment Program (2003), http://www.whirledbank.org/development/sap.html (accessed 9/17/07).

[11] The use of the U.S. dollar as the currency of a foreign country and/or as the currency of world trade.

[12] See http://www.nih.gov/about/hd/strategicplan.pdf and http://ncmhd.nih.gov/ for more about health disparities in the United States and http://www.cdc.gov/syndemics/overview-definition.htm for more information about syndemics prevention approaches.

Chapter 3

What Causes Disease?
Theories of Disease Causation

Whenever I teach my course on ethnomedicine, I always begin the very first day of class by asking the students what they think causes disease. We do a free listing[1] of all the things they can think of, and I write each one on the board. They usually begin with the things with which they are most familiar personally such as infectious diseases like colds and flu, and the current "disease of the year," (e.g., SARS in 2003, avian flu in 2004, west Nile fever in 2006–2007); accidents and injuries; heredity and genetic conditions; cancer, heart disease, and old age; and, most especially, stress.

I always probe about stress: "What is it about stress that makes you get sick?" And they respond by saying that stress affects your immune system and how well you can fight off infection, so if you are really "stressed out," you are more likely to get whatever is going around—especially around exam time and seasonal transitions, or when you are coping with some other emotional or personal issue. Then, free associating, they will often suggest that personal behavior can also cause illness, and we move to a discussion of lifestyle issues such as eating right, maintaining a healthy weight, exercising, using seatbelts, and other preventive behaviors. Moderation is the key. Do nothing in excess. Avoid risky behavior. No sex without latex. Pay attention to prevention. These are the messages of the HMO[2] era. Health maintenance and disease prevention are personal responsibilities achieved by individuals through maintenance of a healthy lifestyle, regular preventive health care, and compliance with necessary medication and treatment to manage chronic disease.

There is usually a lively discussion about whether moderate use of alcohol, tobacco, and other drugs (ATOD) can cause disease—usually the consensus is that only excessive use of these substances can lead to "real" disease (they are beginning to talk about disease as physical pathology here), and that moderate use of alcohol, at least, is not particularly harmful and may even be beneficial according to the studies of the beneficial effects of red wine consumption that they have all heard about (Waterhouse 1995). During discussion of ATOD, there has been a slight shift in the students' thinking, and they ask whether we are talking about disease or illness, because, they assert, that while alcohol may or may not cause actual physical pathology (i.e., disease), it can cause one to be ill (e.g., have a hangover) or uneasy: "like, you might do something you wouldn't have done if you weren't high and that could have all kinds of outcomes—like STD [sexually transmitted disease] or you might get pregnant, or just feel bad—like, I really shouldn't have done that." Here they have begun to think about the differences between disease and illness and have added another aspect, the idea of "dys-ease"—in this case, the feelings of shame and/or regret for doing something "stupid" that may or may not have actual physical outcomes.

Since this is a good point to bring up feelings and emotions, I do: "So," I say, "how do emotions fit in with our ideas about health and illness?" Another animated discussion ensues about whether or not emotions and feelings can actually cause disease. Usually, the students concede that excessive negative emotions (e.g., anger, hate, fear, sorrow, heartbreak, jealousy) could "probably" or "maybe" contribute to the development of physical pathology or exacerbate underlying pathology through the stress response, through the creation of some psycho-neuro-biological-chemical imbalance that can impair the immune system, or through the giving up/given up response (Lovallo 1997, McElroy and Townsend 2004, Selye 1956 and 1976, Webster et al. 2002). It is here that they bring up things they have read or heard that support the idea that feelings can cause disease—for example, that widowers are more likely than married men to die in the year following the death of their wives (Sheldon 1998), or that excessive fear plays a role in voodoo death (Sternberg 2002), or the recent debate over whether the long-term effects of discrimination can affect the health of minorities over and above the negative effects of poverty on their health (Harrell et al. 2003, Ibrahim 2003, Karlsen and Nazroo 2002a, b, Krieger 2001). We explore the idea of poverty as a cause of disease and illness a little more, talking about how poverty can affect health directly because of insufficient resources for decent quality food, shelter, and medical care and indirectly, both through the chronic stress and worry associated with deprivation and economic instability and through the additional emotional stress of discrimination.

"What about anger?" I say. This usually triggers a discussion about violence—both interpersonal violence (beatings, homicide, rape, child abuse, elder abuse) and violence between groups of people or nations (gang warfare, genocide, civil war, war, terrorism). Violence can result in trauma, injury, and death for individuals, but they ask: "Is this really disease?" Are individuals who have been subjected to violence sick or diseased? Or are they just traumatized? By this point the group is fairly clear that they are thinking about disease as some physical, organic, usually measurable, pathology or abnormality of the body and illness as the experience of disease by the patient. Disease is physical and individual; Illness is psychological, personal, and social.

"What about more positive emotions?" I ask. "Joy, happiness, love, fulfillment?" According to the students, these do not "cause" disease or illness. Rather, they are felt to be protective against illness and, perhaps, against disease. Sometimes someone suggests that love might cause illness. After all, you can be lovesick or heartbroken. Most of the students, however, don't think that love is a sickness or that it causes illness.

Since our Western, biomedical system does not usually attribute primary disease causation to emotions, most students are pondering this idea seriously for the first time. "Everyone" knows that emotions affect your "stress level" and can make you feel bad or good, but linking these everyday emotions to short- and long-term health is a new idea for them. In popular culture, in the self-help movement, and in many ethnomedical systems, however, the connection between emotion and illness was made long ago. Just what is the impact of emotion on disease—really? They want to know. I tell them that this is a hot research area at the moment. Scientists are looking at psychological-biological-neurological links between the brain and the immune system and have shown that stress can affect the regulation of the production of stress hormones that, in turn, regulate the immune response (Sternberg 1997, Webster et al. 2002, Wein 2000). Even newer research suggests a mechanism by which stress can accelerate aging in cells (Epel et al. 2004). Thus, knowledge about the biological, physiological, and psychological pathways from stress to disease is unfolding at a rapid rate. It has been estimated that between 50 and 80 percent of diseases worldwide have stress-related origins (Healthy People 2000, WHO 1993a).

After the topic of stress and disease has run its course, I ask again: "What else causes disease?" At this juncture, the class has often become somewhat quiet. They are thinking. So, I wait for them to collect their thoughts. "I'm not going to tell you. There are more. What else causes disease?" "Well, how about the environment?" someone says. They start talking about environmental disasters like the *Exxon Valdez* oil spill,[3] the nuclear disaster at Chernobyl,[4] and the chemical plant explosion in Bhopal, India,[5] and then natural disasters (e.g., earthquakes, floods, tornadoes, and hurricanes) like the tsunami that hit

Asia in 2004[6] and Hurricane Katrina that devastated New Orleans and other gulf coast areas in 2005,[7] global warming, and the vagaries of the weather (i.e., too hot, too cold). "A lot of old people die when it gets really hot and humid here in the summer . . . and all those people died in France last summer (2003) when it was so hot."[8] Then they discuss the impact of difficult environments on health—like mountainous regions and the effects of cold, snow, ice, and high altitude; deserts and their lack of water, intense heat—or cold, and dryness; tropical forests and their snakes, insects, wild animals, and difficult terrain; and large bodies of water—oceans, lakes, rivers. They also list radiation, pollution, pesticides, occupational exposures to hazardous materials, impure water, poor sanitation, and toxins in the environment and in the food supply. Inevitably, someone will ask: "What about genetically engineered food? Or all the antibiotics used in raising cows and chickens?" "And so many people now have allergies and asthma." "And we use so many drugs now, and they can have side effects, so even though they might be necessary for treatment they can hurt you. . . . We just seem to take a pill for everything." Here, the students are beginning to think about how we affect our environment through the technology we use every day, and that our interference with nature can have unpredictable long-term outcomes and unexpected results.

"Is there anything else you can think of?" I ask. In some classes sin will be volunteered as a cause of illness or disease and the role of God in using disease to punish or to test a person. In other classes I have to probe for spiritual or supernatural causes of disease or illness. This leads to a discussion about religion, sin, and breaking moral rules. Since most of the students at my university in New England are Protestants or Catholics, they focus on Christian and Biblical understandings of the role of God, Satan, and sin in health and illness. The idea of possession by the Devil is almost always mentioned and with it, the movie, *The Exorcist* (1973, Warner Studios), which, although old, still seems to be a primary source of information on this topic. Temptation by the Devil and Devil worship are also discussed, although few students actually "believe" literally in the Devil or in witches. Voodoo, which has been the subject of many popular books and movies, is frequently volunteered as a cause of disease and even death in the societies in which it is practiced, but the students agree with the scientific explanation of voodoo death (i.e., auto-suggestion and an extreme stress response, Lovallo 1997) rather than in any supernatural power at work. All of the anthropology majors have read at least one ethnography that dealt with witchcraft or sorcery,[9] and suggest that, like voodoo, witchcraft "works" because the victim believes it does. I suggest, only half-joking, that litigation is our modern form of witchcraft.

"Anything else you can think of?" I ask. Sometimes they might venture some of the "old country" beliefs that they have heard about from their relatives or read about in other courses—evil eye, for example, or *empacho.*[10] Ghosts are sometimes volunteered tentatively as potentially causing problems for people, not disease necessarily, but certainly stress. I then add to our list some of the more common supernatural causes of illness and disease throughout the world that they have not thought of or were not familiar with at all—magic, spirit possession, soul loss or soul theft, gods or spirits, angry ancestors, and fate. "Anything else you can think of?" I ask for the last time. The students say no.

After we have exhausted all of our thoughts, I ask the students to start thinking about how we can group all of these things that we think cause disease or illness according to what they have in common—a kind of typology of disease causation. We identify four domains from our free listing exercise: (1) the individual person and his/her body and personal behavior; (2) the natural world, including the technologically constructed world; (3) the social and economic world; and (4) the supernatural and spiritual world (see Figure 3.1).

Essentially, we have come up with Foster and Anderson's classic typology of disease causation that recognizes (1) the patient or individual, (2) the natural world, (3) the social world, and (4) the supernatural world (Foster 1976, Foster and Anderson 1978, Foster cited in Bannerman et al. 1983). Most ethnomedical systems tend to emphasize either the first two, the individual body and the natural world, or the last two, the social and supernatural worlds, in their underlying theories of disease causation. Those emphasizing the body and the environment tend towards *naturalistic* explanations of disease and illness, and those emphasizing the social and supernatural tend towards *personalistic* explanations.

PERSONALISTIC AND NATURALISTIC DISEASE CAUSATION

In naturalistic explanations, the causative agent is thought to be impersonal, and disease is explained in systemic terms. The body and its physiological systems are upset or put into disequilibrium in some way due to natural causes (e.g., malnutrition, infection, trauma, imbalance in hormones, complications of pregnancy, cancer, etc.). Illness is thought to be an internal, systemic process in which the body reacts to some threat from the outside, natural world. Biomedicine and the humoral medical systems such as Traditional Chinese medicine, Ayurvedic medicine, and homeopathy tend toward naturalistic explanations of disease and illness. The goal of treatment in such systems is the restoration of the normal equilibrium of the body, which is seen as the healthy state. Treatment in naturalistic systems usually entails

Individual Body and Behavior	Natural World	Social and Economic	Supernatural and Spiritual
Genetic makeup	Natural	Poverty	God
Body constitution	environment	Violence	Sin
Immune system	Climate	Terrorism	Breach of taboo
Personality	Technology	Racism	Violation of rules
Risk behaviors	Toxins/pollutants	Warfare	
Lifestyle	Radiation		Witchcraft/sorcery
	Disasters		
Aging			Gods*
Natural processes	Microorganisms		Spirits
gone awry	Insects		Ghosts
	Reptiles		
Accidents/trauma	Birds		Soul loss
	Mammals		Fate
Emotions			
Stress	Plants		
Violence			
	Food, water,		
Hygiene	sanitation		
Malnutrition			

* Italics indicate items usually not volunteered.

Figure 3.1   Typology of Students' Theories of Disease Causation.

the use of medications, diet, exercise, rest, treatment of trauma, and with the advent of biomedicine, a whole host of new medical technologies, surgical procedures, and pharmaceutical drugs.

In personalistic systems, on the other hand, explanations of disease and illness tend to be regarded as the result of direct aggression against the victim through the will or power of some other being, either human or supernatural (e.g., sorcerer, spirit, god). Thus, each patient requires an individual narrative explanation for why he or she became ill. Although there may be actual pathology (from a biomedical perspective), the cause is not located in the natural environment, or natural body processes, but rather in a disharmony in the person's relationship to the social or supernatural world. Treatment in personalistic systems usually entails the restoration of harmony by assuaging the supernatural agent and exhorting or persuading it to restore health or countermanding spells and hexes of witches and sorcerers.

Although most ethnomedical systems are neither purely naturalistic nor purely personalistic, each system tends toward disease/illness explanations at one or the other end of the spectrum. Biomedicine, our Western ethnomedical system, is at the extreme of naturalistic explanations, barely allowing social, spiritual, and supernatural disease/illness causation as possibilities. In biomedicine, every pathology, disease, or dysfunction is thought to have some kind of physical or organic cause or component (even though we may not yet have found it). Biomedicine leaves the spiritual to religion and the supernatural to popular culture. This does not mean that Americans do not search for some ultimate reason for suffering and may even attribute misfortune to the will of God, to fate or luck, or to our own misbehavior, but we tend to explain disease/illness in naturalistic terms and we retaliate against the disease causing agent or attempt to ameliorate the impact of the pathology. In fact, the students who shared their ideas about disease causation were quite skeptical of spiritual and supernatural disease causation and offered scientifically plausible explanations for their apparent effect in other societies (e.g., the stress response) and among the extremely religious in their own society (e.g., belief in God).

At the other end of the spectrum, lie ethnomedical systems like that of the Waorani, a group of tropical forest hunter/gatherer/horticulturalists in Ecuador with whom I have done fieldwork. Traditionally, among the Waorani, every illness or misfortune was believed to be caused by witchcraft, and there was no concept of a natural death. All deaths were the result of witchcraft or homicide and required vengeance against the witch who sent the disease or the people who killed the victim, and often their relatives as well (Erickson In Press, Robarchek and Robarchek 1998). Much as biomedicine ignores the supernatural, the Waorani ignore the natural. This does not mean that the Waorani do not recognize that things like snakebite and influenza are natural phenomenon, but rather that they explain their occurrence in personalistic terms. The disease or misfortune was caused by the witch; therefore they retaliate against the suspected witch or a member of his/her family.

Both naturalistic and personalistic systems are internally consistent and seek to cure or heal by attacking the cause of the disease or illness. In the modern world, biomedicine and many CAM systems are known and available at some level to almost everyone in the world (e.g. through pharmacies, primary health care, WHO immunization programs, etc.). Where personalistic theories of disease causation prevail in the local ethnomedical system, biomedicine is often used in conjunction with the traditional therapies that address the supernatural cause. Biomedicine is used to treat the material disease, what Foster (1983) calls the *proximate* operational or immediate cause of ill health. The *efficient* or ultimate cause, however, is still the human or supernatural agent, and this aspect must be treated before the individual can be restored to health. Similarly, where naturalistic systems prevail, many patients also seek spiritual relief from their suffering through religion and prayer or increasingly through one or more of the more holistic CAM therapeutic systems that treat both body and mind (e.g., yoga, meditation, New Age shamanism).

Joan Engebretson (1998) highlights the basic dualism in Western philosophical thinking that can be seen in Foster's ideas about personalistic and naturalistic medical systems. For Engebretson, the duality lies in "the world of concrete material substance versus that of thought, ideals, and spirit" (Engebretson 1998:37). Figure 3.2 is an adaptation of her model for thinking about healing systems. The model has two axes, the material–nonmaterial and the positivist–metaphysical. According to Engebretson: "The most sensory-based objective material-ist approach to knowing is on the left side of this model, with the most subjective, abstract personal, intuitive, or revealed form of knowing on the right" (1998:39). In this schema, biomedicine would fall into the upper left-hand quadrant, securely within the positivist/material pole. Christian faith healing would fall into lower right-hand quadrant. Catholic exorcism rites would fall into the lower left quadrant and the healing rituals of the Ju'hoansi of the Kalahari Desert that involve night-long rituals of dance and music would fall into the upper right (McElroy and Townsend 2004). Engebretson's model is useful for think-ing about similarities and differences in the myriad different healing systems, theories, and therapies and their philosophical roots.

COMMON THEORIES OF DISEASE CAUSATION IN NONBIOMEDICAL SYSTEMS

Although the students in my classes are always able to expand on the more materialistic, positivist, and naturalistic theories of disease causation that are the basis of biomedicine, they are usually far less able to provide the range of common social and supernatural theories of disease causation found throughout the world. Yet, one of the most pervasive concepts about health in the postmodern world is "a lingering faith in a causal system outside science" (Blaxter 2004:36). Nonbiomed-ical theories can be categorized into six broad domains: balance, body beliefs, the natural world, breach of conduct, malice, and the supernat-ural (see Figure 3.3). It is to these other theories that we now turn.

Body Balance

The idea of balance in the body is basic to many healing systems in which health is conceived as an equilibrium state of the body both internally and in relation to the environment in its physical, social, and/or spiritual dimensions. Illness results from an imbalance or a blockage resulting in too much or too little of some substance or force (e.g., body humor, harmony in relationships, qi). We see this concept in biomedicine in diagnostic tests that assess deviations from the normal composition of body fluids such as blood, urine, hormonal levels, and cholesterol, to name only a few. Therapy involves restoring balance in these humors or substances in the patient.

	Treatment Modality	Positivist ←→ Metaphysical			
		Mechanical	Purification	Balance	Supranormal
		Biomedicine ←→			*Ju'hoansi rituals*
Material ↑	Physical manipulation	Surgery	Cupping	Polarity	Drumming Dancing
	Applied or ingested substances	Pharmacology Pharmaceuticals Herbals	Purgatives Chelation	Humoral medicine	Hallucinogens Aromatherapy
	Energy	Laser/radiation	Bioenergetics	Tai Chi Acupuncture	Healing touch Laying on of hands
	Psychological	Mind-body Psychotherapy Counseling	Self-help Confession	Mindfulness	Imagery Psychic healing
↓ Nonmaterial	Spiritual	Religious participation	Forgiveness Penance	Meditation	Prayer Religious ecstasy
		Catholic exorcism ←→			*Christian healing*

(Adapted from Engebretson 1998:38)

Figure 3.2   Engebretson's Model for Thinking about Healing Systems.

The theory of body balance contains an implicit preventive strategy of moderation in living. Excesses of food, drink, temperature, work, fatigue, and emotion are to be avoided since they undermine the body's equilibrium, and its internal or external harmony. Thus, the prescription for a healthful life in these healing systems is to do all things in moderation. Humoral systems of medicine with their emphasis on moderation and balance prescribe lifestyles for health maintenance, much as does the biomedical specialty of preventive medicine today.

Hot-Cold Balance

One of the most pervasive health concepts around the world today is the hot-cold theory of disease causation, a belief thought to derive from ancient Greek, Arabic, and East Indian traditions (Foster 1953, Logan 1972, Rubel and Haas 1996, Weller 1983). It is common in Asian and Mediterranean cultures and also in Latin America. In the hot-cold belief system, health is achieved through maintaining a balance of hot and cold in the body. Disease is caused by an excess of hot or cold. The body is exposed to hot and cold in two ways—internally through the consumption of food and drink and externally through physical activity, exposure to the elements, and interactions with other people (Goldwater 1983). Maintaining balance is a dynamic process that an individual must undertake throughout the day by eating the right balance of hot and cold foods, avoiding excessive temperature changes (e.g., not drinking cold water when overheated), and avoiding heightened emotional states (e.g., excessive anger or envy) in order to maintain balance, and hence, health. Although hotness and coldness are ascribed to foods, objects, body states, emotions, diseases, and medicines, it is important

Body Balance	**Breach of Conduct**
Hot-cold, humoral	Transgressions
Energy	Breach of taboo
Excessive emotions	**Malice**
Body, society, spiritual, natural world	Aggression (physical and psychological)
Body Beliefs	War and genocide
Blood	Homicide
Organs	Witchcraft
Pollution and contagion	Sorcery
Ingested substances (food, drink, drugs)	**Supernatural World**
Sex	Fate, luck
Heredity	Astrology and horoscope
Old age	God, gods
Natural World	Demons
Accidents	Spirits
Forces of nature (weather, seasons, winds)	Ghosts
Plants and animals	Soul loss or theft
Insects and parasites	Spirit possession

Figure 3.3   Common Theories of Disease Causation in Nonbiomedical Systems.

to understand that actual temperature is not always a factor in such assignment, and with regard to food, neither is spiciness (Scrimshaw 2001). Thus, the hot-cold ascriptions can be either thermal or metaphorical. In Latin America where the hot-cold syndrome has been studied in many different countries, there seems to be no underlying principle for the assignment of existing hot-cold labels nor can the label assigned to a new food item or medicine be accurately predicted (Goldwater 1983).

Although the particulars of what is hot and cold can vary substantially and hot-cold classifications are locally determined, the underlying theory is the same. When a hot-cold imbalance is serious enough, it can shock the system and cause disease. Therapy involves restoring the balance between hot and cold, and usually consists of dietary and herbal remedies guided by the theory of opposites—a cold disease requires a hot remedy and vice versa (Scrimshaw 2001).

Balance of Energy

Another common concept within the body balance paradigm involves the idea that blockage of the free circulation of some substance thought to be vital to life can cause disease. In Chinese medicine, the free circulation of vital energy, called qi, is the life force that animates the body, the energy that allows life. Manipulation of acupuncture and acupressure points is used to release the blocked energy. Therapeutic touch and Christian healing attempt to harness the energy within another person or group of people and direct their combined healing energy to a patient either through prayer, as in Christian healing, or through direct touch as in the laying on of hands or therapeutic touch. This additional healing energy is added to the patient's own weakened energy in order to help him/her recover.

Excessive Emotions

Another very common idea throughout the world is that excessive emotion can cause illness to the self or to others. The person who experiences strong emotions is out of balance, immoderate, and out of control and this can cause illness to the self or to others directly or indirectly.

- **Anger.** Strong feelings of anger, hatred, sorrow, fright, jealousy, envy, and even love can lead to illness or death. In Latin America a nursing mother's excessive anger can sour her milk and place her infant at risk of illness. Social hatred born of prejudice can also cause illness and trauma (e.g., the Holocaust, ethnic cleansings in Rwanda, Bosnia and Croatia, and the Sudan).

- **Sorrow.** Excessive sorrow is also thought to make a person vulnerable to illness. In Western cultures, there is a pervasive lay belief that people can die of a broken heart.

- **Fear.** A sudden fright, called *susto* in Latin America, can result in soul loss, a dangerous condition in which the soul becomes detached from the body and can cause illness or death if not retrieved by the appropriate rituals undertaken by a *curandero/a* (healer) or shaman (Rubel 1964). The sustained fear experienced by physically abused women and children worldwide can lead to mental health problems (e.g., posttraumatic stress disorder, anxiety disorders, depression) in addition to their physical injuries (American Medical Association 1999, Coker et al. 2002).

- **Envy and Evil Eye.** Feelings of envy can result in the casting of the "evil eye" either wittingly or unwittingly, and the envied person can become ill as a result (Scrimshaw 2001). The evil eye entails the belief that a person, who is not otherwise evil, can harm people, children, livestock, or crops simply by looking at them with envy and praising them. The person who gives the evil eye is not necessarily even aware that he/she has the ability to do so, and in this sense is not deliberately trying to cause illness (Dundes 1981). In Latin America, children are thought to be particularly susceptible to the evil eye (Goldwater 1983). Today, the evil eye is widely distributed from India to Europe within the Indo-European and Semitic cultural traditions (Dossey 1998). Talismans, amulets, and charms are worn to ward off the evil eye (e.g., red cord, coral, hamsa hand, eye amulets).[11]

- ***Love and Jealousy.*** In many cultures, passionate love and jealousy are thought to be a sicknesses (Jankowiak 1995). Literature, music, opera, theatre, novels, poetry, and popular media (movies, television, self-help books, magazines, Internet) the world over are replete with stories of the perils of love and love lost (e.g., illness, death, madness). A great deal of magic and witchcraft worldwide is practiced in the service of passionate love. World markets and the Internet[12] are filled with potions, amulets, spells, and fetishes to attract and keep the object of one's desire.

Balance between the Individual and the Social, Natural, and Spiritual Worlds

In some ethnomedical systems, health is envisioned as harmony between the individual and his/her social, natural, and spiritual world. Illness results from an imbalance in any of these relationships. The indigenous cultures of North America exemplify the inclusion of the natural world into their theories of balance and health. Among the Navajo, for example, the maintenance of harmony between man, nature, and the supernatural beings is paramount (Kunitz 1989). To be out of harmony in any of these relationships is to be ill. Healing rituals employ chants, sweats, and sand paintings to restore the individual to harmony with the natural and supernatural world.[13] Native American philosophies and healing practices (especially shamanism) have become popular with the New Age movement[14] whose adherents are seeking a way to reconnect people to the natural and supernatural world (Melton 1995).

Body Beliefs

Enthnomedical systems are enmeshed in cultural beliefs about how the body should look (e.g., size, shape, clothing, decoration), what the boundaries of the individual body are (e.g., for issues of personal space, see Hall 1969), what the inner structure of the body is like, and how the body is believed to function (Helman 2004). Beliefs about the organs and the blood are particularly important in some nonbiomedical traditions.

Organs

Many cultures metaphorically associate illnesses with specific organs or body parts. For example, grief is often expressed as pain in the heart (Good 1977, Good and Good 1981). The Hmong associate mental health with the liver, which is thought to be the site of a person's feelings and personality (O'Connor 1995:92). The uterus, or womb, is the site of much concern worldwide because of its association with childbearing.

Blood

Beliefs about blood and health are widespread. Some belief systems regard blood as irreplaceable and finite. Therefore, any loss of blood is regarded as dangerous. Other systems view an overabundance of blood as a cause of disease and use bloodletting techniques in therapy. Blood viscosity is also thought to vary. Dominicans, for example, believe that blood is like gravy—thin when one is in a humoral hot state and thick when in a cold state (Quinlan 2004). African American lay beliefs hold that blood needs to be balanced regarding its location and volume (high/low), speed (fast/slow), purity (pure/impure, good/bad), and viscosity (thick/thin). Hexing can cause the blood to have abnormal inclusions of magically sent "animals." Blood that is out of balance or that has been hexed requires a remedy (Snow 1993).

Menstrual blood is thought to be dangerous or polluting in many cultures, particularly for men (Buckley and Gottlieb 1988). There are often elaborate methods of avoiding contamination, which can range from the total seclusion of women during menstruation, as in the use of menstrual huts by the Dogon of Mali, West Africa (Strassmann 1999), or the prohibition of cooking, sexual intercourse, and religious duties among menstruating Hindu women in India (Mandelbaum 1970). In rural Jamaica, a woman can use her menstrual blood to "tie" a man to her by putting a little bit of it into the food she serves him (Sobo 1992).

Pollution and Contagion

Pollution and contagion are also common themes in nonbiomedical health beliefs, and there are many sources of pollution that can cause illness. Proximity to a corpse is often considered dangerous and polluting. The Navajo assiduously avoid corpses, graves, and anything connected with death, including archaeological sites and the dwellings of people who have died, to prevent ghost sickness (Kluckhohn and Leighton 1962, Kunitz 1989). Among Hindus in India, many things are sources of ritual pollution—birth, death, food, sex, and even physical contact with castes formerly called the "untouchables"—and require ritual purification (Mandelbaum 1970).

Ingested Substances

The substances that people ingest can also be a source of illness. According to Scrimshaw (2001), food can cause illness through its hot/cold state; by being eaten at the wrong time of day (e.g., eating "heavy" food at night); when it is spoiled, dirty, or raw; and when the wrong foods are combined. The consumption of tabooed foods is a common theory of the cause of illness. People in special states, such as pregnant and lactating women or men about to leave for a hunt, are often forbidden certain types of foods for defined periods of time. Such foods are considered dangerous respectively to the developing fetus, the quality of the mother's milk, or the success of the hunt. Many religions proscribe certain types of foods altogether (e.g., Judaism and Islam forbid pork).

Excess use of alcohol is considered a source of illness in many societies. Addiction to alcohol, tobacco, and other drugs (e.g., heroin, cocaine) is almost universally considered to be dangerous and to produce many social and health problems. Ritual use and sometimes use of less concentrated forms of these drugs are acceptable in many societies. For example, indigenous high-altitude peoples in the Andes chew coca leaves for their stimulant effect similar to that of caffeine, and many psychotropic drugs are used in religious (e.g., peyote in the Native American Church) and healing ceremonies (e.g., *Ayahuasca*, a powerful hallucinogen used by shamans in Amazonia[15]) without negative effects. In pre-Colombian America, tobacco[16] was and today still is considered a sacred plant by many native groups in the Americas, and it is still widely used in sacred, divining, and healing rituals without addiction (Dobkin de Rios 1996, Singer 2004).

Sex

Sexual intercourse (or the lack of it) is also thought to be a source of disease and illness in many societies. The potential of sex to cause illness can be linked to the natural world (e.g., gonorrhea, HPV, overindulgence), to transgressions of social norms for mating (i.e., sex with a forbidden person), or both. The HIV/AIDS epidemic is only the most recent of the life-threatening sexually transmitted infections (STIs) that have plagued the world. Although HIV is a naturally occurring virus that can attack any human, moral overtones have been linked with its acquisition in the United States because of its first appearance among homosexual men and its subsequent spread into other stigmatized groups (e.g., intravenous drug users, commercial sex workers, minorities, and the poor) and finally to the general population (Heymann et al. 1990). In the 19th century, syphilis was similarly stigmatized as a disease related to immoral or intemperate sexual behavior (Magner 2005). In other countries with different social customs surrounding sexual behavior, STIs carry no such moral overtones but are, rather, simply misfortunes.

In many parts of the world parental adultery is thought to cause child illnesses. Incest is thought to lead to mental illness in many cultures. In India, too much sex is thought to weaken men through loss of semen (Scrimshaw 2001). Women in some societies are believed to have sex with ghosts, demons, or the Devil and to suffer illness (especially mental illness) as a result. Violating postpartum abstinence is often thought to result in harm to the infant. Indulging in sex before a hunt or battle is thought to impair a man's strength and to compromise the endeavor. On the other hand, sex in moderation and with the appropriate partner is deemed to be important to health in many medical systems (e.g., Ayurveda, biomedicine).

Heredity

Heredity is widely recognized as a cause of health problems. Some illnesses have long been known to "run in the family" (e.g., hemophilia among the British royal family).[17] Mental illnesses like depression[18] and schizophrenia[19] are now known to have a genetic component.

Young and Old Age

All societies recognize the vulnerability of infants and the inevitability of death and the natural decline in health and mobility among the aged. Newborns, in particular, are viewed as especially vulnerable. The neonatal period (less than 28 days) is considered the most vulnerable period for infants due to largely unpreventable conditions such as birth defects (heart, lung, brain and central nervous system), chromosomal abnormalities, and complications of pregnancy or delivery.[20] In recognition of the fragility of infants, in many cultures children were traditionally not named until they reached one year of age.

Old age is also a time of vulnerability to diseases and the natural degeneration that accompanies the aging process. In some cultures, the aged were hastened to their deaths through socially appropriate suicide (e.g., Inuit [McElroy and Townsend 2004]) or murder (e.g., perhaps the Waorani [Erickson In Press]).

The Natural World

The natural world can be a source of danger to humans. Accidents are obvious causes of trauma and death as are natural disasters such as floods, earthquakes, tornados, hurricanes, and so forth. Change of seasons and unusual variation within a season (too hot, cold, wet, dry) are also thought to cause illness (e.g., flu season). Winds are commonly associated with elevated risk of illness and misfortune. In southern California, the Santa Ana winds,[21] which blow from the desert (the usual winds blow from the ocean inland), are thought to cause everything from homicidal behavior to allergic reactions. Similarly, the Scirocco,[22] warm or hot winds from Libya and Egypt that flow northward into the south-central Mediterranean basin, are blamed for ill health and high seas.

Plants and Animals

The plants and animals of the natural world can cause illness both literally and metaphorically. Many plants are poisonous if eaten, are hallucinogenic if taken internally, can cause skin rashes with contact, or have thorns and spines that can scratch and puncture the skin. Plants can also heal, and many healing plants and herbs are held in high esteem. Most cultures have a long tradition of using plant and animal substances for both prevention and healing, and many modern pharmaceutical drugs are based on herbal medications.[23] Herbal medicines have been documented for centuries in the great medical traditions.[24] Later, herbals (books of herbal remedies) were published in Europe and the United States for common use. Today, the Internet is a vast repository of herbal information and commerce.[25]

The animal world can also be dangerous to humans both instrumentally and metaphorically. Dangers are posed to humans from large mammals such as lions, tigers, and bears; reptiles such as poisonous snakes or crocodiles; birds that carry diseases (e.g., chickens, ducks); amphibians such as frogs and toads; smaller biting insects (e.g., bees, wasps, mosquitoes) and spiders; and down to invertebrates such as worms (e.g., hookworm, roundworm); and finally to microbial and fungal infections. Animals are also thought to cause illness and/or healing metaphorically. They can be a signal of danger or hope, changing the fortunes of those who happen upon them. Our own cultural beliefs in the black cat as a symbol of bad luck; the robin as the harbinger of spring, hope, and renewal; and the snake as the embodiment of the fall from grace in the Garden of Eden are examples of this.

Insects and Parasites

Stinging or biting spiders and insects are also feared creatures both for their annoyance and their potential lethality. Many insects, worms, and smaller creatures (e.g., fungi, bacteria, viruses) can interfere with agriculture, and thus have the potential to cause famine through destruction of crops (e.g., a plague of locusts) or to cause illness in humans. Lice, tics, and parasitic worms have been long-time companions of human beings. Illness due to microbes not visible to the naked eye was attributed to other, usually supernatural, causes, but their environmental associations did not always go unnoticed (e.g., malaria associated with foul smelling swampy areas in Italy, see Magner 2005).

Breach of Conduct

In most cultures, bad behavior (however locally defined) is thought to invite illness usually through punishment by supernatural forces or deities, although sometimes meted out by other humans. Illness is widely thought to be punishment for transgressions and breaches of taboo related to the core activities of human existence: sex, reproduction, sustenance, and death.

Birth is also a dangerous time, and failure of parents to adhere to customary behaviors and taboos surrounding pregnancy, childbirth, and breastfeeding can cause lasting problems, particularly for the child. Many aspects of procuring and consuming food (e.g., hunting, planting and harvesting, food preparation and consumption) are surrounded by taboos, the breaking of which can result in illness and misfortune.

Finally, in most cultures, improper respect for the dead can cause misfortune among the living. Culturally inappropriate treatment of a corpse (from mutilation to improper funerary rituals) can cause problems for both the deceased, who may not be able to pass on to his/her place of rest, and to the living who, invite punishment from the relatives of the deceased (in cases of mutilation), from the ghost of the deceased, or from some supernatural force. Where ancestors are traditionally revered, as in China and Korea, angry ancestors too soon forgotten or not properly honored can be a source of misfortune and illness among their living relatives.

Malice

Aggression of one person against another is an all too common source of illness, injury, and death. Such acts of aggression can be direct and physical (e.g., fights, homicide, or genocide), direct and psychological (e.g., gossip, witchcraft, sorcery), or a combination of both.

Physical and Psychological Aggression

At the societal and interpersonal level, direct physical malice manifests itself in warfare, genocide, terrorism, torture, homicide, and battery. These are all too common occurrences in the contemporary and historical world leading to trauma, death, epidemic disease, starvation, and much psychological suffering (Levy and Sidel 2000, WHO 2002b). Interpersonal violence seems to be part of the human condition. People kill each other for many different reasons—money, property, love, honor, envy, hatred, vengeance—as well as others. Many literary works, television programs, and movies are devoted to murder cases. According to the WHO report on violence, there was one murder per minute worldwide in 2002; more people were murdered than died as a direct result of war (WHO 2002b). The highest rates of homicide in the world are in Africa, South America, and some of the former Soviet states (WHO 2002b).

Gossip, rumor, and slander are used by humans globally to inflict injury on others. Their intent is to alert others to alleged social transgressions (e.g., adultery, excessive drinking, stealing, child beating, etc.) in need of redress. The ruining of reputations surrounding sexual behavior through gossip and rumor is well represented in literature and drama (e.g., Shakespeare's *Othello*, works of Jane Austen) and public life (e.g., the 1998 Clinton–Lewinsky scandal, Prince Charles' adultery). The stakes are often very high for women during their fertile years. Punishment ranges from social ostracism, to the inability to marry, to death. Examples include the witchcraft trials of colonial New England, the killing of women accused of adultery in Greece and other circum Mediterranean societies, and the killing of young women in many Muslim countries for dishonoring their families by having unsanctioned sexual relationships.[26]

Witchcraft and Shamanism

Witchcraft and shamanism are a primary means of harming and/ or healing others in many societies. Witches and shamans are human beings who are thought to have supernatural powers that can both harm and heal. They are believed to be able to transform themselves into animals in order to move about unseen. They can act on their own or their services can be enlisted by other people to inflict harm on another person (usually an enemy), to remove a spell from someone who has been hexed by a witch, or to heal a supernaturally caused illness.

Witches rely on their own insights and inspiration. Witches perform their deeds through both contagious and sympathetic magic. In contagious magic, the witch uses some physical thing that was once in contact with the intended victim—a piece of hair, clothing, or other object. Contagious magic is based on the idea that "things which have once been conjoined must remain ever afterwards, even when quite dissevered from each other . . . whatever is done to the one must similarly affect the other" (Frazer 1940:37). Sympathetic magic, on the other hand, is based on the homeopathic notion "that like produces like, or that an effect resembles its cause . . . the magician infers that he can produce any effect he desires simply by imitating it" (Frazer 1940:11). Thus, the witch uses physical objects that resemble the object or person that the witch hopes to influence. In both sympathetic and contagious magic, the witch uses some kind of spell on the object. This transfers the intended harm to the victim.

Shamans enter the spirit world and enlist the assistance of spirit helpers in their work. They make use of trance and ecstatic states for communicating with spirits who help them in healing and other tasks (Jakobsen 1999, Kehoe 2000). Such trance states can be achieved naturally through the use of drumming and dancing (Siberia), through the use of alcohol (Siberia and Korea), or through the use of hallucinogenic substances (North and South America). Most of the time shamans are working towards positive goals, but many societies recognize that shamans also cause harm. Balikci (1967) described a type of magic (*ilisiniq*) used by Eskimo shamans to bring death or harm to an enemy through contagious magic and the focusing of evil thoughts on the intended victim. In the Americas, shamans cause harm by the introduction of objects (literally or symbolically) into the body of the intended victim. Jívaro shamans of the Peruvian Amazon send *tsentsak* (magical darts, invisible spirit helpers) to pierce their victims and, thus, harm them (Harner 1972). Pomo shamans of the southwestern United States suck out pieces of bone, feathers, or other objects from their patients in order to restore health (University of California Extension Media Center, 1963).

In general, witchcraft and shamanism reflect the intersection of human and supernatural disease causation. It is human beings who cause the illness or misfortune, but they are assisted by supernatural powers or agents in effecting their desires to harm or heal. It is important to note that witches and shamans, like other powerful healers, are both feared and revered and that they are frequently the targets of murder attempts, especially when they are perceived as both powerful and maleficent. Thus, witchcraft and shamanism can be as dangerous to the perpetrators as to the victims. We now turn to the final category of common nonbiomedical theories of disease causation—the supernatural world that operates without the assistance of human intervention.

The Supernatural World

Illness and death are two inescapable aspects of the human condition, and the supernatural world has long been blamed for the many misfortunes that befall human beings. This is not surprising since one of the functions of religion is to explain human pain and suffering and to console those who suffer or grieve. Thus, illness and misfortune have been attributed to the power of many kinds of supernatural beings from one Supreme Being to spirits that inhabit the natural environment as well as to demons, devils, jinni, ghosts, and other supernatural beings that play with humans, sometimes intending misfortune and sometimes causing it only incidentally.

God and Gods

In the major world religions, illness is often interpreted as a punishment. The ancient Egyptian, Greek, and Roman gods caused much misery among the humans who revered them. In Christianity, Judaism, and Islam, the will of God is thought to be an important cause of illness and suffering, and they are interpreted as a test of faith when they seem underserved or as a punishment for sins when retribution is deemed just. Both Buddhism and Hinduism attribute misfortune in this life to bad behavior (i.e., bad karma) in previous lives.

Fate, Luck, and the Stars

For centuries, people in many different places in the world have attributed misfortune, including illness, to fate—a belief that ranges from belief in a pre-ordained life for each person to a more general influence on the life course of the stars and planets based on the time of one's birth (horoscope) and normal astronomical occurrences (e.g., phases of the moon, unusual planetary alignments, etc.,). Astrologers have been consulted for centuries to profile personality and constitutional characteristics and weaknesses and to determine auspicious times for important events (e.g., weddings, building a house, making an important decision, etc.). Historically, China, India, Nepal, ancient Greece and Rome, Europe, and the Middle East all had some variation of this theme. Today, astrology is still very important in China and India and is a booming business in Europe and the Americas where daily horoscopes are printed in newspapers or can be received by phone or online through various Internet sources.[27] Like astrologers, fortunetellers have also been important in many cultures. Fortunetellers use many different methods for divining the future (e.g., reading tea leaves, cowry shells, Tarot cards, the palm). Both astrologers and fortunetellers have advised kings, presidents, and common people alike.

Ghosts, Devils, Demons, Jinni, Spirits, and Others

As discussed earlier, the ghosts of dead ancestors too soon forgotten can cause suffering to the living. Ghosts, in general, can cause illness by proximity (e.g., the Navajo) or through intentional aggression. Devils, demons, and jinni are also thought to cause human suffering and illness. In animistic religions, the spirits that reside in the natural environment and certain places (sun, moon, stars, rivers, lakes, mountains, deserts, caves, animals, winds, etc.) are thought to be the cause of misfortune and illness when they are crossed by unsuspecting humans or when humans do not take proper care of their needs. A host of minor supernatural beings such as fairies, gnomes, trolls, demons, and leprechauns are thought to "play" with human beings for their own amusement, sometimes resulting in misfortune and illness to the unlucky human. It is important to note that in most of these cases (except for ghosts), people are not singled out for punishment for some sin they have committed. Rather, they have broken some rule of engagement with the spirit knowingly or unknowingly (breach of conduct) or were simply in the wrong place at the wrong time (fate or luck). There are two main ways that such spirits cause harm to humans—by stealing their souls and by possessing their body and mind.

Soul Theft or Loss. Soul loss is a common explanation for illness in western Asia and the Americas, to the extent that one is tempted to speculate that it is part of an ancient shamanic system that came with migrants across the Bering Strait. From the Alaskan Eskimo to the Andean Quichua, serious illness is often thought to result when a person's soul has been stolen or lost. In China, as in much of indigenous Latin America, the souls of small children are thought to be only loosely attached to their bodies and may be detached by a fright or by a ghost who enters the body to steal the soul (Potter cited in Foster and Anderson 1978). In soul theft, a spirit is sent by a shaman on his own volition or at the behest of another to steal the victim's soul, thus causing him/her harm intentionally. Another shaman must be enlisted to use his/her spirit helper to find the lost soul in the spirit world and wrestle it back to its owner, fighting the attacking shaman as well if necessary. Elaborate and dangerous rituals are used to find and retrieve the soul, rejoin it to the victim, and restore health.

Soul loss, on the other hand, seems more a matter of fate or luck—being in the wrong place at the wrong time—than a matter of malice. The soul is literally scared out of the body in a syndrome called susto (sudden fright) that exists throughout Latin America and the circum-Caribbean area. The fright caused by an accident or by witnessing a traumatic event (e.g., death of a loved one) can cause the soul to dislodge from its owner causing illness and suffering. Individuals in a weak state (e.g., often children, women, the aged) are particularly prone to susto. In some cases, fright occurs in a place where a spirit resides, for example, a river, and the spirit of the river is blamed for keeping the victim's detached soul from returning. Treatment requires enlisting the aid of a *curandero, espiritista*, or *santero* (spiritual healer) who will coax the soul back into the victim through various rituals and/or appease the offended spirit, thereby restoring health.

Spirit Possession. Spirit possession is different from soul stealing in that the spirit or supernatural being inhabits the body of the victim displacing that person's being and replacing it with his/her own. Possession by a spirit can either cause illness in a victim or be used to heal when a spiritual healer becomes possessed by a powerful helping spirit or deity. The African-based Haitian voodoo complex and other Caribbean religious curing traditions (Santería, Espiritismo) rely on possession of the spiritualist's or priest's/priestess's body to effect healing (Brodwin 1992, Murphy 1995). When maleficent spirits, demons, devils, the Christian Devil, or ghosts possess a lay human, they can cause much suffering and illness. In Espiritismo, a folk healing tradition originally from Puerto Rico, the mere presence of a spirit allows a negative vibration to invade a person and cause him/her to become ill. Cleansing (*dispojo*) with an egg, cigar smoke, special baths and teas, candles, or other ritual items are used by espiritistas to rid a person of these negative vibrations (Singer and Garcia 1989). Among the Jalari in South India, spirits can even possess a child to punish its relatives, extending the social meaning of illness beyond the individual (Nuckolls 1992). Beliefs in spirit possession are geographically widespread (as we shall see in chapter 4).

Multiple Causality

Ethnomedical systems do not tend to maintain a rigid single-cause model of illness. Different kinds of illness are caused by different forces, and even a single illness episode may be seen as having several interacting causes. As Singer and coworkers (1988:378) note, "In the Haitian folk division of medical labor, there are illnesses that are for physicians, illnesses for herbal healers and midwives, and illnesses for spiritual healers. Each type of healer is said to have her own 'territory.'" This statement summarizes the widespread nature of human illness beliefs—multiple causes at multiple levels and the use of many different kinds of medicine and healers depending on the explanatory model for the illness.

CONCLUSION

There is much in the individual body and in the natural, social, and supernatural worlds to cause pain, suffering, and ill health to human beings. The rich variety of explanations for illness presented above attests to the pervasive importance of sickness in human experience and the constant vulnerability that pervades our awareness. Beliefs about illness causation vary greatly but tend to reflect the general understandings of the world found in any given society. Taking all human societies together, we see that, quite literally, almost anything can make you sick, although the range of illness causation beliefs within any individual society is far smaller than this panhuman total. Still, even within a single society, multiple illness beliefs and ways of handling illness can be found. Ultimately, of course, none of us escapes illness and death comes to us all. Most illnesses are self-limiting, but serious illness can lead to loss of social life or separation from the human world in death. The search for the cause, cure, and meaning of illness is the goal of healing systems, which have developed in all times and all places throughout the world. Everywhere "healing requires a legitimated, credible, and culturally appropriate system" (Blaxter 2004:43).

In the next chapter we will take a closer look at the broad patterns of illness beliefs and healing strategies in geographic space and time and the historical linkages among ethnomedicines from disparate parts of the globe.

Notes

[1] Free listing is a qualitative research technique that is part of a series of methods called *systematic cultural assessment* that are aimed at understanding the underlying structure of the domains in a particular area of interest, a kind of cognitive map that shows how people think about a given domain, e.g., causes of disease (see Bernard 2005).

[2] Health Maintenance Organization, a medical care model based on prevention and maintaining wellness and keeping health care costs low.

[3] On March 24, 1989, the *Exxon Valdez*, an oil tanker, grounded on a reef and spilled almost 11 million gallons of crude oil into Prince William Sound in Alaska. http://response.restoration.noaa.gov/bat2/intro.html (accessed 9/17/07).

[4] On April 26, 1986 the nuclear reactor at a power station near Kiev in Ukraine in the former USSR was destroyed, contaminating large areas of three countries with high levels of radioactive elements. http://www.unscear.org/unscear/en/chernobyl.html #Release (accessed 10/5/07).

[5] On December 3, 1984, in perhaps the worst industrial disaster ever, a gas leak from a tank of methyl isocyanate at a Union Carbide plant in Bhopal, India, released some 40 tons of the poisonous gas into the air above the city 8 km. downwind from the plant, killing thousands of people. http://www.american.edu/TED/bhopal.htm (accessed 9/17/07).

[6] A large earthquake on December 26, 2004, under the Indian Ocean hear Sumatra generated giant waves, tsunamis, that crashed on the shores of almost a dozen countries in Asia and Africa killing tens of thousands and destroying homes, businesses, and farms. http://www.npr.org/templates/topics/topic.php?topicId = 1081 (accessed 9/17/07).

[7] Hurricane Katrina hit New Orleans on August 29, 2005, causing more than 1,000 deaths and over $200 billion in damages. http://en.wikipedia.org/wiki/Hurricane _Katrina (accessed 9/17/07).

[8] In June–August, 2003, Europe (from Spain to the Czech Republic and from Germany to Italy) experienced a severe heat wave during which temperatures were 20–30% higher than average, with extreme maximum temperatures of 35–40 degrees Centigrade (95–104 degrees Fahrenheit). France had two weeks of 40-degree weather. Altogether there were about 30,000 casualties in the affected area due to the heat wave. http://www.grid.unep.ch/product/publication/download/ew_heat_wave.en.pdf (accessed 10/5/07).

[9] I teach ethnomedicine both as an undergraduate course in anthropology and as a graduate course in anthropology and community medicine. Most classes are about half anthropology majors and half other disciplines.

[10] In evil eye, certain people are thought to be capable of causing harm to others, especially to children, just by looking at them. *Empacho*, is a gastrointestinal complaint common in many Spanish speaking societies.

[11] Catherine Yronwode's delightful Web site "The Evil Eye" contains pictures of many of these preventive measures and a wealth of in formation on the evil eye (Yronwode 2004), http://www.luckymojo.com/evileye.html (accessed 9/17/07).

[12] A Google search returned 46,500,000 hits for "love magic" and 32,100,000 for "love sick" on January 6, 2006.

[13] See http://www.geocities.com/navajosandpainting/index.html (accessed 9/17/07).

[14] See http://www.religioustolerance.org/newage.htm for an overview of the New Age movement (accessed 9/17/07).

[15] In Quichua, *aya* means spirit and *huasca* means vine. Michael Harner lists as users the lowland Quichua and Zaparo of eastern Ecuador, Jívaro and Conibo-Shipibo of Peru, the Desana, Tukano, and Siona of Colombia, and the Ixiamas Chama/Tacana of Bolivia. (See http://www.biopark.org/peru/Indians-yaje.html)

[16] *Nicotiana rustica, N. attenutata*, and others: http://www.botanical.com/botanical/ mgmh/t/tobacc21.html (accessed 9/17/07).

[17] http://www.geocities.com/jesusib/hemophilia.html (accessed 9/17/07)

[18] NIMH, Depression Research at the National Institute of Mental Health, NIH Publication No. 00-4501, Printed 1999, Reprinted 2000. http://www.eric.ed.gov/ERICDocs/ data/ericdocs2sql/content_storage_01/0000019b/80/19/e0/48.pdf (accessed 10/5/07).

[19] NIMH Genetic Study of Schizophrenia, http://gauss.nimh.nih.gov/sibstudy/ (accessed 9/17/07).

[20] March of Dimes, http://www.marchofdimes.com/home. For complications of labor and delivery, see http://www.marchofdimes.com/pnhec/188.asp; for genetic abnormalities and birth defects, see http://www.marchofdimes.com/professionals/14332_1206.asp; for neonatal death, see htpp://www.marchofdimes.com/professionals/14332_1196.asp (all sites accessed 10/5/07).

[21] http://nrlmry.navy.mil/sat_training/dust/scirrocco/index.html (accessed 10/5/07).

[22] http://www.istrianet.org/istria/meteorology/winds-sirocco.htm

[23] The discipline of ethnobotany addresses native knowledge and understanding of plants and their many uses (see Balick and Cox 1996).

[24] The Vatican Library is a repository for many of these ancient texts. See http:// www.ibiblio.org/expo/vatican.exhibit/exhibit/g-nature/Botany.html (accessed 9/17/07) to view pages from several of the most famous in their collection.

[25] A Google search for "herbals" on 10/5/07 resulted in 2,250,000 hits including everything from historical information to purveyors of herbal medications.

[26] In 1990, Iraq issued a decree allowing men to kill their wives, daughters, or sisters for engaging in adultery. http://www.webcom.com/hrin/magazine/july96/muslim.html (accessed 9/17/07). Such honor killings often occur in societies in which women are treated as property and are punished for proscribed sexual behavior, ranging from pre-marital sex and adultery to flirting and immodest dress, and in some cases having been raped. http://news.nationalgeographic.com/news/2002/02/0212_020212_honor killing.html (accessed 10/5/07).

[27] A Google search of "astrology" on 10/5/07 resulted in over 30,000,000 hits.

Chapter 4

The Geography of Disease Causation Theories

To understand the cultural patterning of theories of disease causation among contemporary groups of people, a large piece of what we call cultural competence in health care in the West today, it is very useful to be aware of the broad geographical differences in the primary organizing features of medical beliefs in the ethnographic past.[1] In chapter 1 we discussed these organizing principles—theories of disease causation, preventive and curative strategies, health care practitioners with special knowledge and training, and a system for care and payment of healers. In chapter 2 we learned about the kinds of medical systems and healers that are typical of different kinds of social organization and subsistence strategies. We learned that healing strategies are likely to be informal at the least complex societal levels (e.g., hunting and gathering groups, nomadic herders, horticulturalists) and that they become increasingly more elaborate and structured at the more complex societal levels (e.g., peasant, state, and global societies). In chapter 3, we discussed many beliefs about the causes of illness and disease, which are held by human beings throughout the world. In this chapter, we will look at theories of disease causation situated at the intersection of geographic and ethnographic space and time.

We first build upon the base provided by the previous chapters to describe the kinds of medical systems that existed around the globe in the ethnographic past, bearing in mind that there has always been contact between different cultural groups over time and space. In this geographic characterization of medical systems, the basic pattern of theories of disease causation are described across broad ethnogeographic areas—ideas that persist to a greater or lesser degree among people of these same cultural groups wherever they reside in the world today. The final section of this chapter turns to a general overview of the geography of contemporary ideas about illness and healing gleaned from more recent studies.

THEORIES OF DISEASE/ILLNESS CAUSATION IN THE ETHNOGRAPHIC PAST

In 1980, George Murdock published an important survey of the geographical distribution of theories of illness using a sample of 139 societies from six areas based on linguistic affiliation and geographical proximity—Sub-Saharan Africa, Circum-Mediterranean (North Africa, Near East, Europe), Asia (India, Pakistan, Tibet, Nepal, Southeast Asia, China, Mongolia, Korea, Siberia, Japan), Oceania (Australia, New Zealand, New Guinea, Indonesia, Polynesia), North America, and South America. This sample includes some of the best documented societies in the ethnographic record. Although such cross-cultural studies using older ethnographies are currently out of fashion in cultural anthropology,[2] Murdock's book remains a rich source of information about theories of disease causation.

Murdock identified two underlying theories of disease causation—*natural* and *supernatural causation* (see Table 4.1). Theories of natural causation included *infection* (invasion by noxious organisms), *stress* (exposure to physical or psychic strain), *organic deterioration* (aging, organ failure, hereditary defects), *accident* (unintended physical injury), and *overt human aggression*[3] (willful infliction of bodily injuries on another human being). Theories of supernatural causation included three subcategories: *mystical causation* with four specific causes—*fate* (ascription to astronomical influences, individual predestination, or ill luck), *ominous sensations* (potent dreams, sounds, sights, etc.), *contagion* (contact with polluted object, substance or person), and *mystical retribution* (violation of taboo or moral injunction); animistic causation with two specific causes—*soul loss* (voluntary or involuntary departure of the soul from the body) and *spirit aggression* (direct hostile, arbitrary, or punitive action of some malevolent or affronted supernatural being); and magical causation with two specific causes—*sorcery* (aggressive use of magical techniques by a human being either independently or with the assistance of a shaman) and *witchcraft* (voluntary or involuntary action of a person believed to

Table 4.1   Prevalence of Theories of Disease Causation in Murdock's World Sample of 139 Societies.

Theory	Important	Mentioned	Total Mentioned	% of Societies Mentioning
Natural Causation				
Total societies mentioning ≥ 1 natural causes			101	75%
Infection (N = 127)	1	32	33	26%
Stress (N = 133)	3	71	74	56%
Organic deterioration (N = 134)	0	29	29	22%
Accident (N = 135)	0	38	38	28%
Supernatural Causation				
Total societies mentioning ≥ 1 supernatural cause			139	100%
Mystical				
Societies mentioning mystical causes (N = 136)			121	89%
Fate (N = 135)	1	28	29	21%
Ominous sensations (N = 135)	0	37	37	27%
Contagion (N = 136)	1	48	49	36%
Mystical retribution (N = 139)	5	105	110	79%
Animistic				
Societies mentioning animistic causes (N = 139)			137	99%
Soul loss (N = 135)	1	32	33	25%
Spirit aggression (N = 139)	118	19	137	99%
Magical				
Societies mentioning magical causes (N = 139)			131	94%
Sorcery (N = 139)	73	46	119	86%
Witchcraft (N = 139)	27	27	54	39%

have special power and propensity for evil). Altogether, these 13 natural and supernatural causes of disease and illness map nicely onto those we discussed in chapter 3, although they do not capture ideas about body balance and life force that are prominent in the great medical traditions.

All of the 139 societies attributed illness causation to at least one supernatural cause and 75 percent of them to at least one natural cause. The most often mentioned supernatural causes were spirit aggression (99%), sorcery (86%), and mystical retribution (79%). The most frequent natural cause was stress (56%).

Regional Variations

Murdock found a different patterning in theories of disease causation by region (see Table 4.2).

Table 4.2 Theories of Disease Causation by Geographical Region.

	MURDOCK'S REGIONS					
	Sub-Saharan Africa	Circum Mediterranean	Asia	Pacific Islands	North America	South America
Primary Causes of Disease in the Ethnographic Past	Mystical retribution Spirit aggression Sorcery Witchcraft	Spirit aggression Witchcraft Evil eye Sorcery Mystical retribution	Spirit aggression Sorcery Mystical retribution Fate	Spirit aggression Sorcery Mystical retribution Contagion	Sorcery Spirit aggression Mystical retribution	Spirit aggression Sorcery Mystical retribution

	CONTEMPORARY REGIONS				
Additional Illness/ Healing Theories	Africa	Europe, North America, Australia, New Zealand	Middle East	Asia	Latin America (Latino and African-American)
Major Medical Traditions	Biomedicine	Biomedicine Osteopathy Chiropractic Homeopathy Naturopathy	Biomedicine Unani Islamic medicine	Biomedicine Ayurvedic medicine TCM Unani medicine	Biomedicine
Body balance	Hot/cold Body, nature Order/disorder	Humoral balance (Greek, Islamic, early European)		Balance (energy; doshas, yin/yang)	Humoral (hot/cold)
Religious healing	Islamic prophetic medicine Traditional African medicine	Christian healing Spiritism Prayer	Islamic prophetic medicine	Islamic prophetic medicine Buddhism Confucianism Taoism Shinto	Spiritism Espiritismo Macumba Vodun Christian healing
Other	Evil eye	Evil eye	Evil eye	Evil eye	Evil eye
Culture-bound syndromes (examples)	Brain fag Zar	Anorexia nervosa Bulimia nervosa	Nerfiza	Amok Koro	Nervios Susto/espanto Pibloktok

- **Sub-Saharan Africa.** Sub-Saharan Africa ranked high in theories of mystical retribution (96%); spirit aggression (96%), and sorcery (78%).[4] Witchcraft (39%)[5] was important in over one-third of the African societies. Evil eye was found only on the northern border close to the Circum Mediterranean region where it is most prominent. Contagious magic (a sorcery technique) was used to cause illness. Ancestors were particularly important as spirit aggressors, but spirit possession was rare. Violation of sex and etiquette taboos[6] was a more important cause of supernatural punishment than in other regions. One or more natural causes of illness were mentioned in 71 percent of the African societies.

- **Circum Mediterranean.** The Circum Mediterranean ranked highest in witchcraft theories—mentioned in 85 percent of the societies and rated as important or very important in the majority (58%). Evil eye was found in 88 percent of the societies in this region but was unimportant elsewhere. Spirit aggression was a main cause of illness in 92 percent of the societies, and the spirits in this region tended to be major gods or deities rather than lesser deities, animistic spirits, or ancestors and ghosts. Sorcery and mystical retribution were lowest here. Breach of taboo was not salient as a cause for mystical retribution as it was in Africa. Fate was moderate in importance. The majority of societies in the Circum Mediterranean region (68%) mentioned one or more natural causes of disease.

- **Asia.** Every society in the Asian sample reported spirit aggression as a major cause of illness and 95 percent mentioned sorcery. Spirits or demons were the primary aggressors rather than gods or deities, which were unimportant. Witchcraft was not particularly important in the region, and sorcery and mystical retribution played only a moderate role. More than half (53%) of the societies in this region mentioned fate as a cause of illness. All but one society included in Asia mentioned one or more natural causes (97%).

- **Pacific Islands.** Spirit aggression was an important cause of illness in this region (92%). There was also a high incidence of sorcery (88%) through spells and exuvial magic (i.e., hair, nails, etc., used in spells), a form of contagious magic, but very little witchcraft (6%). Mystical retribution was not pronounced as a major cause of illness, but was mentioned in 88 percent of societies in the area that has a reputation for many taboos. About three quarters (74%) of societies in the Pacific Islands mentioned natural causes.

- ***North America.*** Sorcery was more important in North America than in all other regions. All of the North American societies reported sorcery, and it was rated as important for most (83%) of them. Object intrusion and presumptive poisoning were the main techniques used by North American sorcerers. Spirit aggression was almost universal (99%) as was mystical retribution (92%). Spirit possession, however, was less important here than elsewhere. Natural causes were mentioned by about two thirds (68%) of the societies in North America.

- ***South America.*** Spirit aggression was very important in the South American region, ranking important in 91 percent of the societies and mentioned by all. Ghosts were important sources of spirit aggression. Sorcery was also important, second in ranking to North America as a major cause of illness and mentioned by 86%. The techniques employed by South American sorcerers were different, however, and included primarily soul theft and spirit aggression. Natural causes were mentioned in 65% of the societies in the South American sample.

In sum, the geographical patterns of illness causation that emerged from Murdock's data reflect the ubiquity and dominance of supernatural over natural causes in the societies included in the sample. All of the societies mentioned one or more supernatural causes. The natural causes of disease were much less prominent than the supernatural causes. Only in Asia and the Pacific Islands were they ever reported as important causes of illness. The ubiquity of supernatural causes of illness might be interpreted as an artifact of anthropologists' interest in the more exotic theories of disease causation, but to me, it seems rather to indicate the fundamental idea that supernatural causes are the ultimate assignment of illness causation in the ethnographic past, and perhaps even today.

This summary of Murdock's work provides the foundation for understanding the geography of theories of illness causation in the contemporary world. To it we add concepts from the great medical traditions that have diffused widely over centuries of interaction among the peoples of the world and the current theories of disease causation that have persisted or evolved and characterize large geographic areas. With the massive exploration and colonization of the East and the South by the West from the 16th century on, the disease causation theories and treatment strategies that began in Greek medicine were spread to most of the world. Although biomedicine enjoys worldwide dominance, it increasingly shares the stage with other forms of complementary and alternative medical systems. Today we live in a globalized, interconnected world—a world that is being reshaped yet again by postcolonial, neoliberal economic policies, the explosion of electronic information and communication technologies, and massive global population redistribution. The world today is a far smaller and much more interconnected place than it was in the ethnographic past (50–100 years ago) or even two decades ago.

CONTEMPORARY TRENDS IN THEORIES OF DISEASE CAUSATION

This section begins with a discussion of the West and the development of the many alternative and complementary medical systems that characterize this region today because the West has been so influential throughout the world, for better and for worse, over the last four centuries. Then a discussion of Africa, humanity's home continent, follows. Because of the slave trade and the forced migration of many Africans to the New World, African ideas about illness and healing have become very important to healing traditions in the Americas. The third area to be addressed includes the Hispanic, Afro-Caribbean, and indigenous healing traditions of North and South America. Next, we look at perhaps the least studied region with respect to ethnomedical beliefs in recent years, the Middle East. The fifth major area is Asia followed by the Pacific Islands. The chapter concludes with a discussion of culture-bound syndromes, those illnesses in different cultures that during the latter half of the 20th century seemed not to conform to biomedical disease categories.

Contemporary Western Societies, the Abrahamic Religions, and Biomedicine

The West is best thought of as Western Europe and its former English-speaking colonies. According to Huntington (1996), the West includes the primarily Roman Catholic and Protestant countries of western and central Europe, the United States and Canada, and Australia and New Zealand. These areas share a common system of values that were influenced by the European Renaissance, Reformation, and Enlightenment. Biomedicine is the dominant medical system in the West. It is the legacy of scientific, rational theory—a medical system based on scientific principles and methods.

The Abrahamic Religious Tradition in the West

Judeo-Christian traditions dominate religious beliefs in the West. Practitioners believe in one supreme God, although in Christianity, the triumvirate of God the Father, Jesus the Son, and the Holy Ghost is mystically woven together into the Trinity, a tripartite concept of God. To this, Catholicism adds the Virgin Mary, the mother of Jesus, and also the pantheon of saints as agents of help and comfort in time of need. Thus, for spiritual assistance, all—God, Jesus, Mary, and the saints—can be entreated to alleviate suffering. The position of other supernatural beings (e.g., angels, the Devil, cherubs, ghosts) in the West is officially downplayed although contested, and many people believe in their power to affect human lives for better or for worse. In the West, healing through prayer and supplication is an important complementary strategy to biomedicine, especially among practicing Christians. In Judaism, as well, prayer and the blessings of a *tzaddik*[7] can be complementary healing strategies (Green 2003).

Christianity first developed as a sect of Judaism around 30. Islam, founded in 622, is the third major world religion[8] with historical connections to both Judaism and Christianity.[9] These three religions are called the Abrahamic religions because of Abraham, the patriarch of the Israelites and Arabs. All three are monotheistic religions, believing in only one God, although the Christian Trinity and use of icons is a departure from the fierce loyalty of Judaism and Islam to monotheism and a ban on any representations of God. All three believe that humans are the highest creation of God. People must read the word of God in the scriptures, must accept God's commandments for living (concern for others, service to others, and social and ethical behavior), and will be rewarded or punished according to how they live. All three religions prohibit murder, lying, and stealing and follow the "Golden Rule": doing to others what we wish others to do unto us. All three religions foster modesty, moderation, and honest work. In return for what God has given, believers must submit to the will of God and glorify Him. The Torah (Old Testament) and the Talmud (a collection of stories, laws, medical knowledge, and moral debates) are the major texts of Judaism; the Bible (Old Testament and New Testament [the teachings of Jesus]) is the main text for Christianity; and the Qur'an (God's final revelation to human beings as revealed to Muhammad) and the Hadith (the sayings of Muhammad) are the main texts for Islam.

All three religions believe that God communicates with people through Prophets. Moses is highly revered by all three traditions.[10] Jesus was rejected as a Prophet by the Jews and Muhammad was rejected as a Prophet by the Christians and the Jews. All three were originally proselytizing religions, although Judaism abandoned this path when the intense persecution of the Jews was initiated. Although these religions share a common historical root and core set of values, they have been unable to coexist peacefully. The disagreement over the status of Jesus and Muhammad led to the fierce competition between Islam and both Christianity and Judaism that has been the source of much war, death, genocide, and suffering over the last two millennia. The importance of an all-powerful God as both punisher and redeemer has influenced the illness and healing traditions of the West tremendously. The ultimate cause of illness and misfortune is God. Thus, although humans can try to alleviate illness, pain, and suffering, only God can take them away.

Biomedical Competitors in the West

In order to fully understand the complexity of medical traditions in the West today, it is also important to have some knowledge of the healing traditions that were in competition with biomedicine in the 19th and 20th centuries, which biomedicine eventually came to dominate, but which are experiencing resurgence under the Complementary and Alternative medicine (CAM) movement today.

Unorthodox Christian-Based Notions of Illness and Healing. In addition to the many established, orthodox Christian religious traditions, there are other traditions that build on the basic premises of Christian belief, but diverge from more general Western belief systems regarding the role of religion in healing. One of these is Christian Science, founded by Mary Baker Eddy (1821–1910) who melded metaphysical healing through thought and the use of the mind with Christianity. According to Eddy the universe is a perfect thought from God and therefore only illusion. Since there is no matter and only mind, illness has no physical reality. Healing occurs through correcting misconceptions about the nature of existence and through spiritual power (Baer 2001, Schoepflin 1988). Christian Science healers pray for the spiritual elevation of their patients so that they will understand the illusion of existence and hence be healed.[11] Today there are about 2,000 Branch Churches and Christian Science Societies in over 80 countries around the world with headquarters in Boston.

Spiritualism[12] is based on the work of Swedish scientist Emanuel Swedenborg (1688–1772) and German physician Franz Mesmer (1734–1815). Swedenborg, while in trance, talked with spirits who described to him a series of spheres through which each spirit would progress as it developed. Mesmer is famous for developing the technique of hypnotism that induced trance states that could facilitate human contact with spiritual beings. American Spiritualism was developed in the 1840s by Andrew Jackson Davis (1826–1910) who claimed to have channeled Swedenborg's spirit to continue his work. Davis lectured while in trance, and these lectures became the basis of a book about the relationship between the spirit and material worlds.

A version of spiritualism that has had great influence in Latin America and the Caribbean was developed in France in the 1850s by Allan Kardec (1804–1869) who viewed spiritualism as a science of the spiritual realm. Kardec extended Christian beliefs to include a spirit world inhabited by eternal spirits who are constantly evolving toward perfection through reincarnation (voluntary, short-term, periods in the material world). These spirits are always interacting with humans and can communicate with them, but some human beings are more adept at spirit communication than others; they are called mediums (people who can channel spirit communication). Modern Spiritualists believe that a spirit world coexists with the material world, and that when a person dies, the soul moves into the spirit world where it will continue to exist and progress for eternity, coming closer to God with each progression. Many spiritualists also believe that the spirits of the dead can communicate with the living through mediums and psychics. Spiritualist healers are mediums who are able to transmit curative energies to diseased parts of the body and to divine the cause of illness through spiritual revelation.[13]

There is little room for supernatural causation or treatment in biomedicine, grounded as it is in the physical, individual body. This split between mind and body makes biomedicine different from all other medical systems that take a more holistic approach to illness and curing. It is at once the source of biomedicine's success in treating the physical and its failure in treating the psychological, social, and supernatural dimensions of illness.

Unorthodox Naturalistic Medicine.[14] There are four nonspiritual healing traditions that developed in the 19th and 20th centuries as competitors to biomedicine that have an important role in health care in the West today. These include osteopathy, chiropractic, homeopathy, and naturopathy. For the most part, they have been sanctioned by biomedicine as complementary and alternative strategies that can be used along with or instead of biomedicine. In particular, osteopathy is considered part of conventional medicine while chiropractic is considered an alternative system. Both, however, have become highly accepted systems for which most health insurance plans will reimburse. The status of homeopathy and naturopathy within biomedicine is less secure.

Osteopathy was developed by Andrew Still (1828–1917) in the American Midwest in 1874. Still believed that disease is caused by problems of articulation (called lesions) in the musculoskeletal system. These lesions produce disordered nerve connections that impair proper circulation of blood and other body fluids. Physical manipulation is necessary to restore the proper articulations. Contemporary osteopaths attend four years of medical school and one year internship. Osteopathy emphasizes the interrelationship of the body's nerves, muscles, bones and organs. Its philosophy is to treat the whole person through the prevention, diagnosis, and treatment of illness, disease, and injury. Today there are 20 schools of osteopathic medicine and some 56,000 Doctors of Osteopathy (D.O.) licensed to practice medicine in the United States, and about 50 other countries worldwide recognize D.O.s.[15]

Chiropractic was also developed in the Midwest by Daniel David Palmer in the 1890s. Palmer believed that disease was caused by disruptions in the "nerve force" (neural transmissions) that were caused by spinal misalignments (subluxations) resulting in dysfunction of the internal organs. Palmer used physical adjustment of the spine to restore the normal nerve force to cure disease. Today, chiropractic is a drug-free, nonsurgical science that treats the whole person paying special attention to the physiological and biochemical factors thought to affect health, including structural, spinal, musculoskeletal, neurological, vascular, nutritional, emotional, and environmental relationships. There are more than 50,000 Doctors of Chiropractic (D.C.) in the United States who are licensed to practice in most states. There are 16 accredited chiropractic colleges in the United States, three in Canada, two in Australia, and one in France.[16]

Homeopathy was developed between 1796 and 1807 by Samuel Hahnemann (1755–1843), a German physician, who thought that disease is caused by a disturbance in the vital or spiritual force that animates the body. To treat disease the physician uses a substance or therapy that produces symptoms in a healthy person that are similar to those caused by the disease (the law of similars). Treatment substances are tailored to the individual patient and used in microscopic doses, the minimal amount to produce the symptom desired (the law of infinitesimals). The goal of homeopathic treatment is to stimulate the body's defense mechanisms and natural healing processes to prevent and treat illness. Homeopathy diffused to North America in the 19th century where it first flourished and then declined, although there appears to be a renaissance of interest in the United States today. Homeopathy is most often used within another health care practice for which the practitioner is licensed (e.g., conventional medicine, naturopathy, chiropractic, veterinary medicine). Homeopathy has been integrated into the national health care systems of Germany, the United Kingdom, India, Pakistan, Sri Lanka, and Mexico.[17] It is also popular in France, Greece, Brazil, Argentina, and South Africa.[18]

Naturopathy originated in Europe and is based on the natural healing practices of four healers: water cures developed by Vincent Priessnitz (1799–1852); water cures and vegetarianism advocated by Theodor Hahn (1824–1883); water cures, diet, and sunlight and air baths used by Arnold Rikli (1823–1906); and Father Sebastian Kneipp's (1824–1897) holistic approach that advocated balance between work and leisure, stress and relaxation, and harmony among the mental, emotional, physical, social, and ecological planes of existence. All of these strategies sought to foster the natural healing process of the body. Benedict Lust (1872–1945) coined the term naturopathy and brought it to North America in 1892.[19] Lust was opposed to the processing of foods because it destroyed their nutritional value and to all drugs and narcotics. The general beliefs that underlie naturopathy include the idea that disease is a response to toxins in the body and imbalances in the patient's social, psychic, and spiritual environment; that nature has the power to cure; and that the body has its own innate healing mechanisms that can be strengthened or stimulated by naturopathic treatment. Naturopathy relies heavily on prevention, education, and personal responsibility of the patient. Naturopathy originally used only hydrotherapy, colonic irrigation (cleansing the entire five feet of the colon), dietetics, and exercise, but many other nonallopathic healing remedies and techniques have been incorporated including homeopathy, herbalism, vitamin therapy, acupuncture, and spinal manipulation.

Today, naturopathy is practiced in Europe, Australia, New Zealand, Canada, and the United States. In Canada and the United States, training for naturopathic physicians (N.D.) includes attendance at a four-year graduate level naturopathic medical school. N.D.s are licensed by 15 U.S. states and the District of Columbia.[20] There are an estimated 4,000 licensed naturopaths in the United States and five accredited schools of naturopathic medicine in North America.[21]

The New Age Movement and Holistic Health. The early followers of these alternative, natural health systems were part of a natural health movement that has evolved into the contemporary holistic health and New Age movements, which include a great variety of healing and spiritual systems (e.g., humanistic and psychosomatic medicine, parapsychology, folk medicine, herbalism, nutritional therapies homeopathy, yoga, massage, bodywork [e.g., Reiki, Shiatsu], medication, martial arts, shamanism, lay midwifery) and their practitioners (Baer 2001).

The holistic health movement developed during the 1960s and 1970s in reaction to increasing dissatisfaction with biomedicine as an impersonal, reductionist, bureaucratic, costly, and dangerous health care system (e.g., drug side effects, over reliance on surgery). It also reflected emerging Green concerns about the destruction of the natural environment and the pollution of the human body with environmental toxins, processed foods, and more recently with genetically engineered foods and the rising concern about lifestyles that are overly dependent on technology. The holistic health movement promotes natural foods and medicines, avoidance of processed foods and pharmaceutical drugs, and less dependence on technology in daily life. The philosophy underlying holistic health, that individuals are responsible for their own lives and for seeking ways to maintain their own bodily and spiritual health and well-being, echoes Western ideals of individualism and self-reliance. The holistic health movement is a widespread, popular movement in the West today, although it is impossible to say how many adherents it actually has.

The West and Indigenous Medicines. There are a great many indigenous populations in the West that include the many different groups of Native Americans[22] in North America (e.g., Navajo, Hopi, Iroquois, Alaskan Inuit), the large group of Maya in Mesoamerica and Central America and other indigenous groups (e.g., Tarahumara in Mexico, the Mayangna of Nicaragua), the large population of Andean Quichua and Aymará as well as the numerous tribal Amazonian groups (e.g., Yanomami, Jívaro, Waorani) in South America, the Sami in Scandinavia, the Samoyed groups in Siberia, the Maori (Polynesian descent) in New Zealand, and the many Australian aboriginal[23] and Torres Straits groups (e.g., Anangu, Koori, Murri).

These indigenous groups are so varied that it is impossible to describe the specific range of medical traditions they encompass in this short book, but a general characterization can be made. For most, if not all, indigenous groups in the West, health is a result of harmony both within the individual and between the individual and the spiritual, social, and natural worlds (Cohen 1998, Parsons 1985, Reid 1983). Sorcery, shamanism, and witchcraft are still important aspects of indigenous theories of illness causation. Indigenous groups also have a long tradition of use of herbal remedies and other empirical techniques for common health problems (e.g., treatment of wounds, bone setting, midwifery).

Contemporary Africa

Africa has regained its continental integrity in my vision of contemporary world regions. While some North African countries (e.g., Morocco, Egypt) are more similar to the Middle East than to Sub-Saharan Africa, the increasing importance of Islam and the decreasing salience of distinct indigenous cultural groups on the continent have reduced the historical importance of the North Africa/Sub-Saharan split that was so important in former times. Except for ancient Egypt, Africa's healing systems until recently were largely oral traditions. What is known about them comes from ethnographies and from the accounts of travelers, missionaries, and explorers. Aside from Egypt and the African kingdoms, most African societies were tribal societies at the time of European contact. Their healing traditions were mostly secret, tied to local religious systems, and passed down through apprenticeship. With colonization came repression of indigenous religion and healing practices, driving them underground. Today, most (estimated at 80% by Bannerman et al. [1983]), Africans rely on traditional healers and herbal remedies and the major theories of illness causation, as in Murdock's analysis, still implicate spirit aggression (from both spirits and ancestors) and witchcraft.

Although Africa is a vast continent and very diverse geographically and politically, there are some basic principles that underlie many traditional African medical systems including: (1) the idea of balance in the physical, psychological, spiritual, and social dimensions; a dualistic model of disease causation that includes both natural and supernatural causation and the idea that a natural disease can be caused supernaturally; (2) the idea of hot/cold opposition and that these opposing qualities are important in disease and cure; (3) the use of ritual incantations or behaviors and trance induced by music, dance, or chanting in curing and healing; and (4) the practice of divination of the cause of illness to assess the psycho-social problems that underlie the disease and need to be addressed for resolution (Frierman 1985, Koumaré 1983). To these Green (1999) adds a set of more naturalistic theories that he calls indigenous contagion theory: (1) harmful organisms that can invade the body and cause illness (e.g., worms, tiny insects), (2) mystical contagion or pollution that can be caused by contact with an impure, unclean, or harmful substance or person, (3) the environment as a source of illness (e.g., filth, illness carried in air or water), and (4) illness that results from a breach of proper behavior or violation of a taboo. Thus, there is a mix of traditional spiritual and natural disease causation theories in contemporary Africa that has not been fully appreciated until recent times, although it was also evident in Murdock's analysis.

Many traditional cultures in Africa are animistic and require the acceptance of a highly structured universe of magical forces that permeate all aspects of life. Many also require adherence to personal obligations within a rigid gender and social structure. Individuals ordinarily see themselves as part of an interdependent group in which competition is discouraged. Thus, illness primarily results from disordered relations between the individual and the supernatural or social world, and healers become the mediators between the patient and the social and spirit worlds.

Many healers are specialists in sorcery and spirit possession, divining the cause of illness, or the removal of ritual pollution. Others specialize in kinship therapy to adjust social relations between spouses, parents and children, siblings, and ancestors. Thus, traditional healers play a powerful role as mediators in the social system. Treatment is aimed at both the individual body and restoration of balance in the patient's relations with the social (family, community) and supernatural (spirits, ancestors) worlds, and a kin-based therapy group is an important part of most treatments. Treatment often involves herbal remedies, medicines, rituals, aromatic plants, fumigation, and sometimes residence with the healer. The goal of treatment is to appease the spirit, ancestor, or witch that caused the illness so that the patient will be left alone by the supernatural entity and thus healed.

In a very real sense, then, traditional African healing practices are aimed at both the bodily and mental states of the patient and are inseparable from local religious beliefs. The patient is treated within the local social, cultural, environmental, and supernatural context; disease/illness and curing/healing are culturally constructed and negotiated in the therapy group. The treatment is tailored to the specific patient in social context. With the growing importance of Islam, Christianity, and biomedicine in all parts of Africa, their healing theories and strategies are increasingly being incorporated into local traditional medical systems.

Contemporary Latin America

Latin America, like Africa, comprises an area that is diverse geographically and politically. It is comprised of Mexico, Central America, the Caribbean, South America, and the large contemporary Latino population in the United States. This area has a shared history of colonization primarily by Spain and Portugal, participation in the African slave trade that fostered current African American and Afro-Caribbean cultures, the presence and displacement of the indigenous populations (e.g., Tarahumara in Mexico, the Mayangna in Nicaragua, Quichua and Yanomami in South America), and the current dominance of Christianity in this region. Thus, for hundreds of years the area has included a mix of indigenous, European, and African populations and their cultural and healing traditions. In contemporary Latin America there are three broad themes that characterize traditional ethnomedical beliefs: (1) humoral—hot/cold—beliefs, (2) spiritism, an African and French influence, and (3) soul loss, a largely indigenous belief. Interestingly, of these, only soul loss is reflected in Murdock's data showing the overriding importance of spirit aggression and sorcery for the indigenous peoples in this region.

Humoral medicine which we discussed extensively in chapter 3 is widespread in Latin America, the Caribbean, and the southwestern United States, which was formerly part of Mexico. Humoral beliefs may have been introduced by the Spanish after the conquest or may have been part of the indigenous Americans' belief systems, many of whom consider the universe to be a system of balanced opposites. Whether introduced, indigenous, or a mixture of both new and old, it is still widespread in the region today. It is important to note that the categorization into hot or cold varies significantly from place to place, even quite locally (Logan 1973) and that actual beliefs in and knowledge about the hot/cold syndrome vary by gender, rural–urban residence, and education. Women, rural residents, and less educated populations are more likely to know about and utilize the hot/cold belief system in their own health maintenance, while it may be a vestigial folk belief among modern, educated, urban dwellers. Nevertheless, it remains an important underlying explanatory theory and has been a persistent organizing belief about illness throughout Latin America for centuries.

Spiritism came to Latin America with the slaves brought from West Africa to Brazil and the Caribbean between the 1500s and the 1800s and developed into its present form within three separate but related religious movements: Macumba in Brazil; Santería, in Cuba, but now widespread in the Caribbean as well as the United States (primarily New York, New Jersey, Miami, and Los Angeles), South America (i.e., Argentina, Brazil, Colombia, Mexico, and Venezuela), and Europe (i.e., France and the Netherlands); and Vodun (Voodoo) in Haiti (see Brodwin 1992, Laguerre 1987, Murphy 1993 and 1995, Olmos and Paravisini-Gebert 1997, Voeks 1993 and 1997, Wedel 2004). All of these complexes involve elements of the religious beliefs primarily of the West African Yoruba, but also of the Ewe, Fon, and Bantu peoples who were brought as slaves to these areas. They have also incorporated elements of other religious traditions, notably Catholicism and Kardecian spiritism. Today, adherents to these spiritist traditions come from all ethnic groups and social classes. The foundation of spiritism includes the following beliefs:

1. There is a spiritual energy or vital force in the world and this vital force is part of all natural and supernatural phenomena.
2. Humans have both a physical and a spiritual body.
3. There is a high God who is the source of the vital force and all life and nature.
4. This high God communicates with the world through spirits that include guardian spirits, ancestors, and nature spirits.
5. Spirits constantly contact the physical world.
6. Humans can be contacted by and can learn to contact, channel and embody or incorporate the spirits (primarily through possession) for healing and spiritual evolution.
7. The role of humans is to keep the vital force that sustains and animates the world moving by praising and nourishing the spirits.

Thus, although humans live in the natural world, they can come into contact with the supernatural world by way of the spirits who can enter the human world at any time. Humans and spirits are always interconnected. Although Macumba, Santería, and Vodun share these basic beliefs, they are all religions with oral traditions, and have many local variations. Each will be described in more detail below.

Macumba is an umbrella term used to refer to three religious traditions that developed in Brazil: *Candomblé*, *Umbanda*, and *Quimbanda*. Candomblé originated in the 16th century as a religion practiced by African slaves. In Candomblé there is a high God (Yoruban Olorum) who is the supreme deity and who interacts with the world through the 50 or so lesser guardian spirits called *orishas*. The orishas have individual personalities, ritual preferences (e.g., songs, dances, foods), and are connected to natural phenomenon (e.g., water, trees, plants, stones). They are constantly contacting humans in the physical world, and humans can learn to contact and incorporate these spirits for healing and spiritual evolution. The orishas must be nourished through human praise and animal sacrifice. Their temples are called houses or yards and each is managed by a high priestess and her "family" (i.e., helpers—not necessarily biological family members). The spirits and Catholic saints can help the priestesses and priests to guide, heal, and assist followers of the religion. The means for enlisting help from the orishas include supplication through prayer, ritual divination (through oracles such as cowry shells or dominoes), and offerings. During Candomblé ceremonies, the orisha can inhabit the body of the priestess/priest through possession and trance during which he/she can "speak" to supplicants to offer advice, guidance, and healing strategies.

The Candomblé ritual has two parts: a private preparation and a public ceremony often called a mass. Only priests and initiates participate in the preparations, which can take a week and involve getting the ceremonial costumes ready, decorating the house where the mass will be held with the colors associated with the particular orishas that will be honored at the mass, and preparing food for the banquet. On the day of the ceremony, divinations are performed and animal sacrifices are offered to the orishas and then cooked for the ceremonial feast. During the public ceremony, the orishas are asked to attend the ceremony and do so by inhabiting the bodies of priests who enter into trance and perform dances that honor the orishas. The leading priest sings songs that recount each spirit's deeds. The mass ends in a grand feast that can last beyond midnight. Other aspects of the rites include the use of African language, music, and dance.

Umbanda began in 1904 as an offshoot of Candomblé. It combines beliefs about spiritism from Candomblé, Catholicism, Kardecian spiritualism, Hinduism, and Buddhism. Its priests communicate with both orishas and with the Catholic saints. Quimbanda began as a variation of Umbanda. In the popular imagination Quimbanda is associated with the darker side of spiritism and the intention to use the spirits for evil ends rather than for good (similar to witchcraft). The main difference between the two, however, seems to be that Umbanda tends to emphasize Christianity more than Quimbanda, which places more emphasis on the complex relationships between humans and spirits. The Christian evangelical movements in Latin America in the last quarter century have been particularly critical of the Afro-Brazilian religious traditions, perhaps an additional reason for Quimbanda's undeserved reputation for black magic. Today, Umbanda and Quimbanda are primarily religions of middle-class urbanites in Brazil, Uruguay, and Argentina. These three religious traditions have come to be seen as three separate religions with common roots, much as the Abrahamic religions discussed earlier have a common root, but have diverged in significant ways from the parent religion.

Santería, which developed among African slaves in Cuba and then spread widely throughout Latin America and the Caribbean, is a combination of Candomblé and Spanish Catholicism. The high God, Olorum, and each of the orishas are associated with a Catholic personage or saint.[24] Early on, these associations of Yoruban deities with Catholic equivalents served to disguise the persistence of African religious practices at a time when slaves were forbidden to practice their own religion. In the 1800s Kardecian spiritualist traditions were brought from France to the Caribbean and incorporated into the African-based systems of spiritism in Cuba to form a new religion, Espiritismo. Today, Santería is a truly syncretic religion with elements of Candomblé, Catholicism, and Karedecian Spiritism whose practice varies locally. The development of Espiritismo in the Caribbean parallels the development of Umbanda in Brazil. The structure and rites of Santería are basically the same as those of Candomblé with temple houses, ritual use of drumming, trance, animal sacrifice, and spirit possession for spiritual and healing purposes.

Vodun (Voodoo, Vodoun, Voudou, Vodon) is another African-based religion found primarily in Haiti. It has been traced to the Vodun religion in 18th century Dahomey,[25] which is still practiced widely in modern Benin. The basic organizing principles and beliefs are the same as those of Candomblé, except that the orishas are called *loa* (or *iwa*) and the structure of the spirit world is somewhat different. In Vodun, the high god, Olorun, is remote and unknowable. A lesser god, Obatala, created the earth and its life forms on Olorun's authority. There are hundreds of lesser spirits (loa)—those that originated in Dahomey called Rada and those added later in Haiti called Petro. These spirits are entreated to help people through offerings of animal sacrifice and gifts. Slightly different from the other spiritist religions, Vodun followers believe that each person has a soul composed of two parts: a *gros bon ange* (big guardian angel) and a *ti bon ange* (little guardian angel). The ti bon ange leaves the person when he/she is possessed by a loa during Vodun rituals. The detached ti bon ange can be damaged or captured by a sorcerer while it is outside of the body. Thus, the priests (*houngans*) and priestesses (*mambos*) are at risk and in danger during their duties of ritual spirit possession. The Vodun temple, called a *hounfour* (a house), has a pole in the center where Olorum and the loa communicate with people. The rituals consist of a feast; a cornmeal drawing (*veve*) unique to the loa for whom the ritual is being performed; drumming and rattling; chanting; dancing by the houngan, mambo, and hounsis (students); possession by the loa; and animal sacrifice (later used in a communal feast for the congregation). Scholars today argue over whether Haitian Vodun is a syncretization of African religion and Catholicism or whether Vodun is a completely separate religion. The controversy may be due to the fact that Vodun is an oral tradition and has many local variations. Many Haitians say they practice both Vodun and Catholicism.

Most practitioners of Vodun limit their activities to white magic, which brings good fortune and healing. However, the undisciplined loa can also be used by sorcerers to perform black magic aimed at doing harm. Another belief unique to Vodun is the belief in zombies, people thought to be resurrected after death and burial, but who have actually been placed under the influence of powerful drugs by a sorcerer who controls their behavior.[26] The practice of sticking pins into effigy dolls as a method of cursing or harming a person seems to have originated in New Orleans. The darker side of Vodun has been exploited in American horror films that overemphasize these rare practices. For the most part, Vodun is like Candomblé, Umbanda, and Santería, all of which enlist the help of the spirits to better human life and health.

Soul loss is a common explanation for illness especially among indigenous groups in the Americas and by practitioners of Vodun. Souls can be lost in a variety of ways—through a fright or traumatic event, because of a weakened state (e.g., disease, grief), being in the wrong place and having the soul enticed out of the body by a local spirit, or by having the soul stolen by a witch, sorcerer, or other spirit. Infants, small children, and the elderly are thought to have weakly attached souls that can easily be lost or stolen resulting in serious illness. Shamans, priests, sorcerers, and other kinds of supernatural healers are enlisted to entice the soul back to the body of its owner by coaxing it back if it has simply wandered away, by convincing the possessing spirit to give it back by appeasing the spirit, or by stealing it back. Elaborate and sometimes dangerous rituals and ceremonies usually accompany attempts to treat soul loss.

In much of Mexico, Central, and South America, it is the *curandero/curandera* (male/female curer), who is sometimes also a *brujo/a* (witch) or a shaman, whose job it is to cure patients of the various natural and supernatural illnesses that afflict them. Curanderismo is not one thing; "it is an art, a calling, a gift" (Torres with Sawyer 2005:4). Thus, each curandero/a emphasizes different aspects of healing (mind/body) and uses different techniques (ritual/herbal/medicinal), combining them in different ways in his/her own distinctive healing strategy. There are, however, some common strategies used by curanderos/as. They usually use herbal remedies and other medicines (pharmaceuticals, over-the-counter preparations, etc.) and provide advice on diet, exercise, and lifestyle for simple physical ills. For more serious problems involving supernatural causes, curanderos/as will often perform a ritual cleansing of the patient or his/her home. Many use some kind of divination to discover the cause of the illness and/or enlist supernatural assistance to resolve the problem. Supernatural assistance often comes from the Catholic saints, God, *La Virgen* (Virgin Mary), and various local indigenous spirits or deities. The curanderos/as can receive assistance from their supernatural helpers in dreams, through objects with ritual power, through trance induced naturally or with hallucinogenic drugs, or through direct communication with the supernatural world (Arvigo 1994, Joralemon and Sharon 1993, Kunow 2003). Ritual cleansing, called a *limpia*, usually involves the symbolic "sweeping" of the body or a place to cleanse it from evil spirits and harm. The curandero/a uses some physical items (e.g., branches of a plant or tree, feathers, an egg, tobacco smoke, alcohol, aromatic water, etc.) to perform the limpia. For more serious illnesses, it might be necessary to have a ceremony with a *mesa* (table/altar) on which various sacred objects are placed. The patient and his/her family (and sometimes the entire community) attend the ceremony in which the curandero/curandera enlists the aid of his/her supernatural helpers and in some cases hallucinogenic substances to cure the patient.

Today, medicine in Latin America is an amalgam of biomedicine, the various CAMs, spiritism, curanderismo, shamanism, and the many folk traditions and beliefs of its diverse populations, which include indigenous peoples and the descendants of European colonists and African slaves.

The Middle East

The Middle East includes the eastern part of Murdock's Circum Mediterranean region that was a result of the east–west divisions after the fall of the Roman Empire and the Christian–Islamic split that begins geographically with Turkey. The northwestern Mediterranean became part of Europe and the West; Turkey and the rest became the Islamic Middle East. Here, Murdock found the primary causes of disease to be spirit aggression, witchcraft, sorcery, and mystical retribution (see Table 4.2). Today, the Middle East area is large and varied with many local health beliefs and folk healers. For more than 1,000 years, mainstream medicine in this area followed the Greco-Arab system now known as Unani medicine (Baasher 1983). The basic principles of Unani are those of Greek medicine, a system based on maintaining optimal balance of humors through diet, exercise, and moderate lifestyle and treatment with medications, bloodletting, cupping, and lifestyle modification. Islamic prophetic medicine is the other major medical tradition in the area and is dependent on faith in Allah and teachings in the Qur'an (see chapter 2). Like Christian healing and biomedicine, Prophetic medicine and Unani have different theoretical bases for understanding illness and for effecting cure (i.e., spiritual vs. physical cause and intervention). They can be used as complementary or alternative strategies depending on the religious views of the patient.

In addition to these well-developed medical belief systems, there are two other main beliefs about disease attribution in the Middle East that lie outside of the more naturalistic explanations of Unani—belief in the evil eye and belief in jinn (pl. jinni). Evil eye, the belief that a person, who is not otherwise evil, can harm people, especially children, simply by looking at them with envy and praising them was discussed extensively in chapter 3 along with methods for prevention and cure. Jinni were briefly discussed in chapter 3 along with other supernatural agents like ghosts, devils, demons, and spirits—all thought to have the ability to cause human suffering. Jinni merit more detailed attention here because they are particular to the Middle Eastern area, to Arab folklore and traditional Semitic beliefs, and to Islam.

Westerners are familiar with jinni (genies) from Arabic folk tales (e.g., *Aladdin's Lamp*) and the popular 1960s television sitcom, *I Dream of Jeannie*.[27] Jinni are thought to have the magical ability to make the wishes of their master come true, always with some unforeseen misfortune since the precise statement of the wish is crucial to its manner of fulfillment. Those who seek aid from jinni are usually faced with deception, and the fulfillment of the wish never quite meets the intent of the original request, but rather reflects the jinn's desire to do mischief if not outright evil.

Jinni are part of Islamic belief. They were created by Allah before humans and are thought to live in a world parallel to that of humans. They eat, marry, have children, and die. They are mostly invisible to human beings, but they can appear in animal or human form. The jinni's power over humans lies in their ability to whisper deceptions that can lead humans to disobey Allah. Jinni can also impart evil eye. Prior to the emergence of Islam, the ancient Semites believed that jinni were spirits of ancient peoples who could make themselves invisible or change shape into animals and were responsible for human disease and mental illness. Thus, belief in the jinni's ability to cause misfortune to humans has a long history in the Middle Eastern area. To fight the jinni, Muslims must seek refuge in Allah—reciting *audhu billah* (I seek refuge in Allah) or other remembrances of Allah.[28]

It is interesting that Murdock found spirit possession, witchcraft, and sorcery to be the main causes of illness in the Middle Eastern area and that the Qur'an forbids (*haram*) sorcery (as well as astrology and fortune telling), but has methods to deal with spirit possession and temptation by the jinni. The parallel with Christianity is clear—witchcraft is condemned, but spirit possession and temptation by a "bad angel" or Satan are still held by some Christians to be legitimate causes of illness or misfortune.

At the end of the 19th century, much of the Middle East came under foreign domination, primarily by France and Britain, and Western medicine was introduced into the region, officially eclipsing traditional medicine in importance until the 1960s when many of the countries in the area, which had gained their independence after World

War II, experienced a resurgence of interest in traditional medicine and herbal medicine (Baasher 1983). Today, medicine in the Middle Eastern countries includes biomedicine, Unani medicine, Prophetic medicine, and the many folk traditions and beliefs of its diverse populations, which include many indigenous tribal groups, Christians, and Jews. A recent editorial in *The Lancet* notes that this area of the world, which was at one time the leader in science and medicine, today is "the most neglected health area in the world" due to the widespread violence, political unrest, and strife there (Editorial 2006:959).

Asia

Like the other areas, Asia is vast and culturally and ecologically diverse. Several distinct world religions (Buddhism, Tao, Shinto, Hindu, Islam) and cultural traditions are found there. The area is bound together by the early influence of China and India in the region and today by the increasing economic influence of China, Japan, Korea, India, Taiwan, and Singapore. The area is so complex that it will be discussed by subregions: East Asia—Japan, Korea, and China; West Asia—India, Pakistan, West Bengal, Bangladesh, and Afghanistan; Central Asia—the former Soviet territories (e.g., Kazakhstan, Mongolia, Siberia); and Southeast Asia (i.e., Burma [Myanmar], Thailand, Cambodia, Laos, Vietnam). Religiously, Pakistan, part of India, Bangladesh, and the many countries in Central Asia are primarily Muslim;[29] Hindus are dominant in India and West Bengal; Buddhism is the primary religion in Southeast Asia; Confucianism, Taoism, and Buddhism in China; Buddhism, Christianity, and Confucianism in Korea; and Buddhism and Shinto are dominant in Japan.

China dominated the eastern part of Asia for thousands of years. The central and western part, mostly desert and steppe areas through which the Silk Road wound its way to the Mediterranean, was fought over by Arabs, Mongols, and the Chinese until the Europeans carved up the whole of Asia and divided it among themselves in the 19th century, introducing biomedicine and Christianity to their new colonies. Much of eastern and southeastern Asia was heavily influenced by Chinese culture and Traditional Chinese medicine; the west by Persian and Islamic culture and medicine; and India and Southeast Asia by Indian culture and Ayurvedic medicine. Alongside the great medical traditions that flourished in the historical classic civilizations and in urban centers of Asia today, however, many smaller, local medical traditions persisted as well. Central Asia and Siberia had altogether different healing systems based on shamanism. Korea also has a strong shamanic tradition.

In Asia, as in much of the rest of the geographic areas studied by Murdock, the main causes of illness were spirit aggression, sorcery, and mystical retribution. Murdock also found that ideas about fate as a cause of illness were moderately powerful in this area as well, particularly in China, Korea, and India, where astrology, fortune telling, and luck are still important concepts in explanations of life events, misfortune, and health and illness. The four major geographic regions of Asia and their contemporary medical beliefs and systems are discussed below.

Eastern Asia

Traditional Chinese medicine (TCM) has long dominated eastern Asia (Kleinman et al. 1975). In China, and in all the places to which the Chinese migrated, it is a major provider of health care. China has made it national policy to integrate Traditional Chinese medicine and biomedicine and to train practitioners of both systems in the important points of the other. The traditional system continues to flourish and develop and has incorporated scientific research methods for testing the efficacy of traditional drugs and therapies. TCM is also the foundation for the development of the traditional medical systems of Oriental medicine in Japan and South Korea. These systems are essentially TCM elaborated by locally available herbal medicines and healing techniques.

In Japan, traditional medicine is known as *kampo* (*kanpō*). It is a variation of TCM that developed over 1,000 years of contact with Chinese healing practice. In modern Japan, where biomedicine has been predominant since the end of World War II, there has been a resurgence of popular and professional interest in kampo therapies that are widely used by the population and are thought to cause fewer adverse reactions and side effects than the pharmaceutical drugs and invasive therapies of biomedicine. Furthering its appeal, kampo was officially recognized and encouraged by the Japanese government in the 1980s (Ohnuki-Tierny 1984). All kampo practitioners must be licensed in allopathic medicine and all licensed physicians can legally practice kampo. Kampo practitioners are thought to spend more time with their patients, listen to them, and treat the problem in a more holistic manner than straight allopathic physicians. About 72 percent of Japanese physicians say they used kampo therapies in their practice, suggesting an emerging hybridization of kampo and biomedicine (Holliday 2003). In addition to biomedicine and kampo, Japanese national health insurance also covers acupuncture, moxibustion,[30] Japanese traditional massage, and *judo* (bone setting) therapy (Holliday 2003).

In South Korea, Oriental medicine (OM) is called *Hanbang*. It is based on TCM but uses Korean herbal medicines. It is the primary health care system for more than 20 percent of the population in Korea. OM focuses more on restorative herbal medicines than does TCM. Its other contributions include *Sasang* constitutional medicine based on personality types characterized by sorrow, anger, gladness, and enjoyment; *Saam* acupuncture, which uses 60 points located below the joints of the arms and legs; herbal acupuncture; and Korean hand acupuncture. There are eleven private OM colleges and about 11,000 registered OM practitioners in Korea. Since 1987, health insurance has covered some OM procedures (diagnosis, acupuncture, moxibustion, some herbal medicines), but for the most part is a private sector, primary-care phenomenon (Holliday 2003, WHO 2001).

Today, Japan and South Korea are among the most developed nations in the world, and they have integrated medical systems that combine both biomedicine and traditional medicine. Oriental medicine is integrated into hospitals, clinics, and training institutions and its practitioners are licensed by the state. Both countries actively promote the use of traditional medicine at the primary and secondary levels of health care and through coverage of some therapies through national health insurance. As in South Korea and Japan, variations on Traditional Chinese medicine are also practiced in the cosmopolitan and highly developed islands of Taiwan, Hong Kong, and Singapore, where they are mostly in the private sector (Holliday 2003).

To understand the nonmedical healing practices in Eastern Asia it is necessary to have some knowledge of the predominant religious systems, because, as we have already seen, religion, medicine, and healing are deeply intertwined phenomena. The major religions of China are Confucianism, Taoism, Buddhism, and traditional Chinese religion (ancestor and spirit worship); of Japan Buddhism and Shinto; and of Korea Buddhism, Christianity, Confucianism, and traditional shamanism.

Confucianism is an ancient ethical system that teaches the values of *li* (ritual, propriety, etiquette), *hsiao* (love and obligations of parents and children), *Yi* (righteousness), *xin* (honesty and trustworthiness), *jen* (benevolence, humaneness towards others), and *chung* (loyalty to the state). Adherents must perform four rituals at important life-cycle events (birth, puberty, marriage, death). Confucianism is often combined with Taoism, their founders having been contemporaries.

One of the oldest and most important of the Confucian classics texts is the *I Ching* (Book of Changes), which describes the ancient system of cosmology and philosophy at the heart of Chinese cultural beliefs. This philosophy includes the dynamic balance of opposites, the evolution of events as a process, and the acceptance of the inevitability of change. It is also a system of divination that seeks to know the future by using 64 hexagrams that represent the states and the dynamic relationships of eight elements (heaven, thunder, water, mountain, earth, wind, fire, swamp). A random method (e.g., tossing coins or dice) is used to select the hexagram and the text associated with it is read and interpreted.[31] Today, the *I Ching* is used in much the same way as astrology, bibliomancy (using randomly selected passages of a sacred text in divination or assistance in solving a problem), and Tarot readings.

Tao means the way or the path. Tao is an energy or power that flows through all things. It regulates natural processes, maintains balance in the universe, and embodies the harmony of opposites (yin/yang). The Three Jewels of the Tao are compassion, simplicity, and patience. Followers of Tao must take care to promote individual health and vitality by nourishing their qi; living a life of compassion, humility, and moderation; letting nature take its course; and seeking answers to life's questions through meditation and observation. Taoists believe that human interference with nature is a primary cause of imbalance in the universe. Like Confucianism, Taoism is more a way of life than a religion and neither religion has a God, gods, or even scripture.

Buddhism developed in what is now Nepal during the 5th century BCE and spread to the Indian subcontinent, Central, Southeast, and East Asia over the next 2,000 years. It is the fifth largest religion in the world today. Buddhism has a number of different traditions, but most of these share a common set of fundamental beliefs. The basic tenet called the *Four Noble Truths* is that life inescapably entails suffering from sickness, misfortune, pain, failure, and the impermanence of pleasure. The cause of suffering is the desire to have and to control things that ultimately cannot be controlled. Buddhism promises an end to suffering in Nirvana, a state of enlightenment and cosmic oneness with Buddha in which the individual is released from attachment to the world when his/her mind is released from the desires that cause suffering.

Following the *Eightfold Path* leads one to enlightenment. This path includes three areas of training and practice: *prajna* (discernment, wisdom) is the heart of Buddhism and teaches that wisdom will come if the mind is pure; *sila* (virtue and morality) teaches that all living things are equal and that people should treat others as they themselves would like to be treated; and *samadhi* (concentration and meditation) teaches the means to achieve the mental development needed to achieve freedom from suffering.

Buddhists also believe in reincarnation and rebirth and that most people go through many cycles of birth, life, death, and rebirth. In reincarnation, an individual may come back as the same person repeatedly, as did Buddha in his many reincarnations. More often, however, an individual comes back as a different entity. It can take many cycles of life and rebirth to release attachment to desire and the self, but finally doing so leads to enlightenment.

As Buddhism expanded across Asia, it split into two main forms, Mahayana and Theravada, that developed independently from one another. Mahayana Buddhism is found in China, Japan, and Korea. The Mahayana tradition places less emphasis on the attainment of enlightenment for all individuals, recognizing that this is time-consuming and not practical for all. It teaches that Buddhists should live in this world while committing to compassion for all, living the rules for a good life, working toward enlightenment, and helping others to attain Nirvana. Mahayana Buddhism is more like a traditional religion in which there are higher beings that can assist people in life and in which people are expected to help each other as well. Since the 13th century, Theravada Buddhism has been dominant in Southeast Asia (Thailand, Burma, Cambodia, Laos). In Theravada Buddhism, the ultimate goal is personal wisdom and achievement of Nirvana. It requires great personal dedication as a monk or nun and commitment to meditation to achieve personal enlightenment. Other variations of Buddhism developed in Japan, Tibet, and Korea. The shared goal of all forms of Buddhism is enlightenment through patient discipline, meditation, right living, and compassion for all life. This is the common core of Buddhist thought and tradition.

It is easy to see how Confucianism, Taoism, and Buddhism were compatible in China. For the most part, they are philosophies of life that are not dependent on belief in a monotheistic God. They embrace both the natural and spiritual world, according reverence to nature and to maintaining balance and harmony in relationships between humans and the natural and spiritual world. They are complementary rather than competing philosophies. As philosophies for living a good life, they complement Traditional Chinese medicine whose fundamental theory relies on the idea of balance, harmony, equanimity, and lifestyle moderation. TCM treatments aim to restore the body to equilibrium and thus reinforce the basic principles of Confucianism, Tao, and Buddhism.

Traditional Chinese religion exists alongside these great religious traditions and includes a wide variety of practices such as ancestor worship, veneration of the many gods and goddesses from Chinese mythology and folklore,[32] veneration of nature (e.g., animals, mountains, the sun, moon, earth, heavens, and stars), fortune telling and divination (e.g., the *I Ching*, Chinese astrology[33]), feng shui,[34] shamanism, and mediumship. It has also incorporated elements from Confucianism, Taoism, and Buddhism. Traditional Chinese worship, legends, festivals, and devotions are associated with ancestors, gods, and goddesses and still form an important part of contemporary Chinese culture.[35] These traditional practices have existed for thousands of years and are accepted as complementary to Confucianism, Taoism, and Buddhism. Traditional Chinese religion, more than TCM and the major religions, addresses the uncertainties, misfortunes, and persistent, serious, or unexplained illnesses that people experience over the course of their lives by attempting to influence the course of fate and appealing to ancestors and spirits for assistance. It is traditional religion that addresses spirit-caused illness and misfortune.

In Japan, the two main religions are Buddhism and *Shinto*. Shinto (way of the gods) is an animistic religion in which the *Kami* (gods or spirits) are part of all life. Shinto developed from a mixture of ancient Japanese practices of nature worship, fertility cults, divination techniques, hero worship, and shamanism. There are four different kinds of Kami: (1) nature Kami who live in natural phenomena, such as stones, rivers, and trees; (2) guardian Kami associated with particular places or clans; (3) people who were exceptional in life and became Kami after death (including the emperors); and (4) Kami who are associated with creative forces. The Kami are led by Amaterasu Omikami, the goddess who is worshipped at the Ise Shrine, the main shrine of Shinto about two hours from Tokyo. Different shrines are dedicated to different Kami, who have their own personalities. The Kami are benign and sustain and help people. They can be asked for assistance through prayers and offerings.

Basic beliefs and practices of Shinto involve ancestor worship, reverence for nature, belief in the sacredness of all human life, reverence for *musuhi* (the Kamis' creative and harmonizing powers), achieving *makoto* (sincerity or true heart), emphasis on the family or group rather than the individual, and preservation of family tradition through birth and marriage rituals. Followers of Shinto emphasize personal cleanliness, and they bathe, wash their hands, and rinse out their mouths frequently. They worship and honor the Kami at their shrines and at home altars. Shrine ceremonies usually include cleansing, prayers, offerings, and dancing. *Omamori* (charms, amulets, talismans) from specific shrines are worn to protect against evil and misfortune and to help in healing. Shinto shrines, such as Ishikiri Shrine in Osaka (associated with tumors) and Nakayama Temple (associated with obstetrics and gynecology), are important sites where people can seek assistance from the Kami for healing in contemporary Japan (Ohnuki-Tierney 1984). Like Traditional Chinese religion and TCM in China, Shinto helps the Japanese deal with the spirit world and with the misfortunes of life while kampo fills the role of TCM treating the physical body.

In Korea, the religious system is a combination of indigenous beliefs and world religions imported into Korea. Thus, Koreans embrace Buddhism, Christianity, Confucianism, and shamanism, and they have developed a new religion called Ch'ondogyo.[36] Perhaps more so than in other East Asian countries, however, shamanism still has a lively presence in Korea. As we have already seen for many areas for the world, belief in a world inhabited by spirits is both widespread and ancient. Shamanism is undoubtedly the oldest form of religion in East and Central Asia and is thought to have prehistoric origins. Korean shamans are similar to those found in other parts of Asia where shamanism has strong roots (e.g., Siberia, Mongolia, northern Japan). Unlike other areas, however, in Korea, most shamans are women. They are sought by people who want the help of the spirit world to overcome problems they are facing in their lives. Female shamans (*mudang, mansin*) hold services (*kut*) to gain good fortune, to cure illnesses, to exorcise evil spirits, to propitiate local gods, spirits, or ghosts,[37] and to guide the spirit of a deceased person to heaven. In some ways, Korean shamanism can be considered a form of traditional medicine since consultations often involve illnesses (physical, psychological, social). The Korean shaman is a professional who is consulted by clients when they need her to manipulate the spirit world to solve human problems. The Korean shaman, as other shamans in Asia, is a master of spirits. In Korea, Oriental Medicine fills the role of TCM in China and kampo in Japan.

Central Asia and Siberia

Shamanism is the preeminent religious phenomenon of Siberia and Central Asia (Jakobsen 1999). Our Western understanding of the concept of shamanism comes from the Tungus people of Siberia where the role of the shaman was that of mediator between the human and spirit world (Eliade 1989, Jakobsen 1999). The shaman is a specialist in the human soul and s/he travels to the spirit world to enlist the spirits' assistance or to do battle with them to alleviate human suffering. S/he has a special relationship to the spirits in which s/he can seek help, power, and knowledge. Shamans engage the spirits by entering their world through an ecstatic magical flight or journey. Shamanic ecstasy, or trance, is a key means of communicating with the spirit world. Shamans develop their own idiosyncratic ways of entering into trance and interacting with the spirit world that vary from place to place.

Western Asia

Ayurvedic medicine is practiced in India, Pakistan, Bangladesh, Nepal, and Sri Lanka. Unani, the Persian medical system based on Greek medicine, is also an important medical system in this area. In most of these countries, Ayurvedic, Unani, and biomedicine are officially recognized, parallel medical systems with little integration among them. In India there are more than 150 undergraduate and more than 30 postgraduate colleges for Ayurveda, and training can take up to five years.

The major religions in Western Asia include Hinduism, Buddhism, and Islam. Ayurvedic medicine reflects the philosophies and practices of Buddhism and Hinduism, while Unani is associated with Islam. Ayurvedic medicine developed alongside Hinduism and Buddhism over the millennia. References to it are found in the oldest Hindu texts, the Vedas.

Hinduism is thought to be the world's oldest organized religion. It has the third largest following after Christianity and Islam. Unlike most other major religions, Hinduism has no single founder. It is based on a number of religious texts developed over many centuries. Its oldest religious texts, the Vedas, predate the Old Testament by about 1,000 years. The four Vedas contain spiritual insights and practical guidance for living as well as hymns, incantations, herbal remedies, and rituals. Other important scriptures include the eighteen *Puranas* (which discuss the creation of the cosmos, genealogies of gods and sages, the creation of human beings, and dynastic history) and the epic poems, the *Ramayana* (which depicts the life of Rama) and the *Mahabharata* (which depicts the life of Krishna). The *Bhagavad Gita*, part of the Mahabharata, is a collection of the spiritual teachings of Krishna and is perhaps the most widely read of the Hindu spiritual texts.

Modern Hinduism incorporates four themes from the ancient Vedic tradition: (1) *dharma* (individual ethics, duties and obligations), (2) *sansāra* (rebirth), (3) *karma* (right action), and (4) *moksha* (salvation). Hinduism, like Buddhism, focuses on self-improvement for the ultimate purpose of attaining enlightenment, oneness with God, and freedom from suffering. Hindus believe that this state of salvation can be attainted by living people through various methods (yogas). In Hinduism, yoga is a spiritual practice whose primary goal is self-realization, not simply the flexibility training familiar to Westerners.

Although Hinduism is often thought by Westerners to have many gods and goddesses, Hindus actually recognize a single god, Brahman: infinite, pure existence and knowledge. However, most Hindus worship God as a less abstract concept in the more personal forms of gods and goddesses. Brahma, the Creator; Vishnu, the Preserver; and Shiva, the Destroyer are the three most prominent personifications of God. Hinduism also recognizes that God can appear to humans under multiple names and in many forms and that sometimes God comes to earth as a human being to help humanity on the road to moksha. Such incarnations of God are called avatars (*avatāra*). Rama and Krishna are among the most famous of Vishnu's avatars. Most Hindus follow one of two major divisions of Hinduism, Vaishnavaism in which Vishnu is seen as the ultimate deity, or Shivaism, which sees Shiva in this role. In rural areas, however, Hindus often worship their own village gods and goddesses. The earth goddess (variously known as Lakshmi, Boodevi, and by other names) is particularly important as she rules over harvests and disease.

The doctrine of karma is intimately related to the realization that all is one. It teaches that everything that a person does leaves an impression in the mind and determines the kind of person one becomes in the future. Good actions develop good tendencies; bad actions lead to bad tendencies that can cause bad things to happen in an individual's current life and also in subsequent lives. Virtuous actions bring the soul closer to God and lead to rebirth with higher consciousness. Evil actions hinder this progression and the soul is reborn as a lower form of worldly life. Over the course of time and many deaths and births, one can strive to purify the mind and intellect, in order to experience God, the end of sansāra, and attainment of moksha.

Most Hindus worship God through images, such as statues or paintings. Worship, called *pūjā*, can take place at home or at a temple. People make offerings of food, water, or flowers and burn incense, light candles, ring bells, or wave a fan to honor God at the shrine at dawn and dusk. Other forms of worship include meditation, chanting God's name/s, and reciting scripture. Worship at temples is not required, but many Hindus go to temples during religious festivals. Each temple has a priest who performs the rituals and ceremonies required to maintain it. Food offerings made to God by worshippers (*prasāda*) are given by the priest to other worshippers, monks and nuns, and others visiting the temple. Eating prasāda is thought to be spiritually beneficial to the recipient.

The chanting of mantras (such as the holy word, *Aum*) helps people to focus on holy thoughts or to express love and devotion for God. Mantras also give courage during hard times and help people to invoke their inner spiritual strength. Vegetarianism, for Westerners a hallmark of Hinduism, is not actually required of Hindus but is embraced by many as a spiritual practice. It is tied to the doctrine of karma and to sansāra, since doing no harm to living things is a basic principle of Hinduism. The similarities between Hinduism and Buddhism are substantial since they share a long history of development in India. Hinduism is one of the most tolerant of all the world religions and has a long history of recognition or incorporation of holy people from other religious traditions (e.g., Buddha, Jesus Christ, Mohammad) because of its underlying philosophy that there are many ways to understand the same truth and to worship God.

Hindus can turn to God, gods and goddesses, and temples in times of illness, but mainstream Hinduism relies less on the idea of illness as a punishment than on illness as the result of lifestyle choices, the same philosophy that underlies Ayurvedic medicine. However, especially among less-educated rural populations, gods and goddesses can cause illness, and spirit possession is a common reason for illness and other misfortune. For example, village gods can be angered by human behavior and send illness, often to a child or some other blameless person, to call attention to the social disharmony that needs to be rectified. Illness will only be resolved if the people involved make the proper changes in their lives. Gods and goddesses can also come to be associated with particular diseases. In Bangladesh, the local goddess of smallpox was an obstacle to the eradication of smallpox in the 1960s and 1970s. The skin eruptions caused by the disease were thought to be a visitation from the goddess and villagers feared immunization because they thought it might offend the goddess.

Spirit possession has been an important cause of mental illness and distress in India. Many forms of physical illness and misfortune have also been blamed on spirits and local gods and goddesses angered by human behavior. Recent research, however, suggests that there has been a shift away from spirit possession by spirits who have names and personalities toward a more homogenous notion of spirits in conjunction with the use of the psychological terms tension and depression to characterize what would previously have been labeled spirit possession (Halliburton 2005).

Finally, fate is also an important concept in Indian notions of the cause of illness and misfortune among humans. It is intimately related to ideas about karma and how people live their lives. Astrology has a strong appeal in India and astrologers are sought out for both general horoscope readings based on place and time of birth (temperament is an important concept in Ayurvedic medicine) and for determining auspicious dates for important life transitions, such as marriages, and other important undertakings, like building a house or opening a business.

Southeast Asia

Southeast Asia has long been influenced by the neighboring Chinese and Indian civilizations whose religious and healing traditions have permeated all of Asia. Ayurvedic medicine has particularly influenced the Buddhist countries of Thailand, Burma, and Laos, while Traditional Chinese medicine (TCM) had a bigger influence on traditional medical practices in Vietnam. While Ayurveda and TCM provide the theoretical basis for much traditional medicine in Southeast Asia, specific medicines and therapies were also developed from the locally available flora and fauna and from preexisting healing traditions of local groups in the area. In addition, as we have seen in other areas, rural populations had their own local healing, often shamanistic, traditions that existed alongside the medical traditions of the urban kingdoms in Southeast Asia. Thai medicine is an interesting example of this process.

There are two distinct medical traditions recognized by scholars of traditional Thai medicine—the royal tradition and the rural traditions that developed among the hill tribes in northern Thailand (e.g., the Karen and Hmong) and among rural peasant farmers. The royal tradition was based on traditional rural practices that had been influenced by Ayurvedic, TCM, and Western medical concepts over hundreds of years of interaction with Indian, Chinese, and Arab merchants and European explorers who arrived as early as 1504. But it was Buddhism, Ayurvedic medicine, and other Indian influences that were especially important to the establishment of the royal medical traditions in the Kingdom of Siam. By about 1600 royal medicine was a coherent and effective health care system that was sustained by the king and the urban elite (Salguero 2003). During the 1800s, King Rama III ordered the inscription of 60 stone tablets with charts of the acupressure points and 1,100 herbal remedies. These were installed on the walls of the temple, Wat Po, along with more than 80 statues depicting yoga postures and massage technique, forming the basis of the Traditional Medical School at Wat Po. Between 1895 and 1907, the temple medical school published several important herbal manuals containing a summary of the ancient traditional lore

preserved there, which are the core curriculum for the school of traditional medicine that still operates at the temple.

In Thai philosophy, life is a holistic blend of three essences—the
physical self (the body), the nonphysical self (emotions, thoughts,
spirit) or mind/heart (*citta* in Thai), and energy, which holds citta and
the body together. The Thai idea of energy is similar to that of qi in Chinese medicine and prana in Indian philosophy and is thought to flow
throughout the body by way of more than 72,000 *nadis* (meridians).
Thus, the Thai, like many other peoples in the Asian area, view illness
as an imbalance of body, mind, and spirit. In Thai medicine, such
imbalances are thought to cause a breakdown of the immune system
and the body's naturally healthy state that leaves the body vulnerable
to a variety of illness and disease-causing agents (germs, allergies,
environment, heredity, emotional, psychological). Thai medicine uses a
holistic approach to healing that addresses physical, mental, and
energy problems simultaneously (Brun 2003). The medical system has
three branches: diet and herbal remedies for imbalances in the physical
body, spiritual healing therapies for imbalance of citta, and Thai massage for imbalances of energy. Spiritual healing blends Buddhist
prayer, meditation, and mantras with and shamanistic healing traditions; Thai massage aims to balance energy and energy flow; and diet
and herbal therapies aim to restore the physical body to health.

Today, Thai massage, Nuad Thai (known in various forms as
Nuad Boran, Thai Massage, Thai Yoga Massage, Thai Yoga Therapy,
sen therapy, etc.), is a particularly well developed therapeutic technique. Thai massage involves manipulation of the patient's body using
passive stretching and gentle pressure along energy lines (sen). *Jap sen*
is the Thai form of acupressure. Massage takes place in a quiet, medi-
tative location, and the practitioner uses both his/her hands and feet to
adjust the skeletal structure, to increase flexibility, to relieve muscular
and joint tension, to stimulate the internal organs, and to balance the
body's energy system.[38] Thai herbalism is based on an underlying
humoral theory of four body elements/qualities (earth/solid, water/liq-
uid, air/movement, and fire/heat) associated with different body organs
and systems that interact with each other. Balance in the elements
results in health and imbalance in disease.

The medical traditions of the hill tribes and rural peasants in
Thailand are less formal than those of the royal medical tradition, but
the underlying philosophy of imbalance is similar. Spirit aggression
(spirit possession, angered spirits, etc.) as a cause of illness is more
elaborated in rural medicine than in the more naturalistic royal medical tradition where spiritual causation tends to be more metaphysical
than personalistic. Actual healing practices among rural healers, however, vary substantially from group to group and even from practitioner
to practitioner. The herbal traditions of rural medicine tend to be secret

and handed down from teacher to apprentice, and practitioners are shamans who use shamanic healing techniques such as exorcisms, amulets, charms, and incantations along with herbal remedies. Because of this secretive tradition, in fact, there have been very few studies of traditional rural medicine in Thailand (Salguero 2003).

The Pacific Islands

The Pacific Island region is also large and diverse, consisting of very different kinds of societies—from the remote archipelagos in the Pacific Ocean to the predominantly Catholic Philippines and predominantly Islamic Malaysia and Indonesia. In the Pacific Islands, the pattern of indigenous beliefs about illness are, as Murdock found, largely based on ideas about spirit aggression and sorcery, although there are also natural causes of illness (e.g., sprains, breaks) that can have an ultimate supernatural cause.

Many larger island nations in the Pacific, in particular the Philippines and Malaysia, have long been influenced by TCM. The Philippines, Malaysia, and Indonesia have also been influenced by Ayurvedic medicine and Hindu and Buddhist traditions of India. As Islam came to these areas, so did its medical traditions. In addition, the Philippines, Malaysia, and Indonesia have their own local herbalists, midwives, and spiritual healers. The Philippines has a significant herbal tradition with over 1,000 known medicinal plants used by *herbolarios* (healers) and *hilots* (midwives). There are also quasi-religious healers, faith healers, acupuncturists, and *medicos* who combine traditional and biomedical techniques in the Philippines. In Malaysia, traditional healing is based on a concept of a vital soul substance called *semangat*, which if depleted can render the individual less able to defend against evil forces and environmental assaults. Traditional Malay healers called *bomoh* use rituals, incantations, and spells to identify illness and to exorcise the spirit responsible for simple illnesses and more elaborate rituals and psychodrama for more serious illness, as well as community-wide rituals for epidemic diseases. They also use herbal remedies and physical therapies like bone setting and massage. In Indonesia, local traditional medical beliefs and healing practices are similar to those in Malaysia. In more remote New Guinea, sorcery, soul loss, and bad behavior are important theories of disease causation, and healing focuses on counteracting the evil power causing the disease and/or strengthening the individual's personal power to overcome it (Kun 1983).

Research in Polynesia, the smaller Pacific islands, atolls, and archipelagos strung across the South Pacific in several different island groups (Soloman Islands, Vanatu, Tuvalu, Wallis and Futuna, Tonga, Western Samoa, Cook Islands, Society Islands) and in Hawaii suggests that the core health belief paradigm defines the normal human condition as one of fragile, easily disrupted equilibrium in the supernatural, environmental, and social systems and within the individual body. Disruptions of equilibrium in any of these systems can cause disease, and the cause must be found and treated. In Hawaii, for example, traditional healing involved seeking forgiveness and reconciliation from the offended person or spirit through sacrifices and offerings to reestablish equilibrium and harmony (Chang 2001). In much of Polynesia, the indigenous spirit world usually included three levels: gods, ancestors, and other spirits. To this pantheon was added the Christian God after contact and conversion by Christian missionaries (Parsons 1985). The kinds of informally trained healers reported in most of the islands included bone setters, masseurs, herbalists, midwives, sorcerers, and healers specialized in treating illnesses caused by different categories of spirits (Parsons 1985). The island inhabitants still adhere to their traditional medical systems and use the introduced biomedical system as a complementary system with the underlying pragmatic view that indigenous medicine treats indigenous diseases about which biomedicine knows little, and biomedicine treats the European-introduced diseases about which indigenous medicine knows little. There is a similar coexistence of beliefs in the indigenous spirits and in Christianity. The two systems accommodate to each other with indigenous systems expanding their ideas about illness and treatment pragmatically to seek that which works best for the specific ailment (Parsons 1985).

The Pacific Islands region is vast and varied, perhaps more so than any of the other regions discussed thus far. As in the other regions, biomedicine is dominant today, but it shares the stage with Traditional Chinese, Ayurvedic, and Unani medicine; with Christian, Islamic, Hindu, and Chinese religious health and curing traditions; and also with other kinds of indigenous healers versed in natural and supernatural healing techniques who are important sources of health care in their communities, especially in the Philippines, Indonesia, Malaysia, and New Guinea.

THE CULTURE-BOUND SYNDROMES

Our tour of the geography of theories of illness causation would not be complete without a brief discussion of what have been called the culture-bound syndromes (Hughes 1985, Simons and Hughes 1985, Yap 1965, 1969a, 1969b). These are a group of syndromes that anthropologists have come across in the different cultures that seemed not to correspond to any known biomedical diseases or mental disorders. They were described by Hughes as "unfamiliar ways of being crazy" (Hughes 1985:3). The current DSM-IV defines a culture bound syndrome as "[a] recurrent, locality-specific pattern of aberrant behavior and troubling experience that may or may not be linked to a particular DSM-IV diagnostic category. Many of these patterns are indigenously considered to be 'illnesses,' or at least afflictions, and most have local names" (American Psychiatric Association 1994:844). Today, anthropologists understand them as culturally *defined* syndromes that reflect an insider's way of describing, understanding, and interpreting a set of locally recognized symptoms (Scrimshaw 2001). The current approach to such culture specific disorders in biomedicine and psychiatry is to treat them as mental health disorders (i.e., as variations of anxiety, depression, somatoform disorders, or adjustment disorders, attention-seeking behavior, and feigning illness) that have locally elaborated symptoms. Neither the current DSM-IV nor the International Classification of Diseases, 10th edition (ICD-10) includes culture-bound syndromes separately from other mental illness (WHO 1993b).

According to Simons, they are "local ways of explaining any of a wide assortment of misfortunes" (Simons 2001). Thus, in addition to being local variations of recognized psychiatric conditions, they also represent what anthropologists call "idioms of distress" (specific illnesses that occur in some societies that are recognized by members of those societies as expressions of distress). The syndromes are not bound to a particular culture, but rather are "related to special sociocultural emphases or stress situations that can occur in very diverse societies" (Jilek 2001:7). I discuss several examples of culturally defined syndromes by geographic area (see Simons and Hughes 1985).

- **Africa.** In West Africa, brain fag is a condition experienced by students. Its symptoms include difficulty concentrating, remembering, and thinking; it can also include head and neck pain, pressure, tightness, blurring of vision, and feelings of heat or burning. In North Africa and some parts of the Middle East there is a condition called *zar* in which the victim believes he/she is possessed by a spirit. Symptoms include dissociative episodes with laughing, shouting, hitting the head against a wall, singing, or weeping. Individuals may show apathy and withdrawal, refusing to eat or carry out daily tasks, or may develop a long-term relationship with the possessing spirit.

- **The West.** In North America, Europe, and Australia, *anorexia nervosa* and *bulimia nervosa* are culturally defined syndromes that may overlap. In anorexia there is severe restriction of food intake that is associated with a morbid fear of obesity and distorted body image. Excessive exercise may also be used to lose weight. Bulimia is characterized by binge eating followed by purging through self-induced vomiting, laxatives, or diuretics and a morbid fear of obesity. Today anorexia and bulimia are increasingly being seen outside of this region.

- **Middle East.** *Nerfiza* (nerves) is a culture specific-disorder found in Egypt, northern Europe, Greece (*nevra*), and Mexico and Central and South America (*nervios*). It is characterized by common, often chronic episodes of extreme sorrow or anxiety that induce somatic complaints such as head and muscle pain, nausea, appetite loss, insomnia, fatigue, and agitation. It is more common among women than men and has been linked to stress, anger, emotional distress, and low self esteem.

- **Asia and the Pacific Islands.** These locations have several prominent culture-specific syndromes. *Amok*, found in Indonesia and Malaysia, is an indiscriminate, seemingly unprovoked episode of homicidal or highly destructive behavior that is followed by amnesia or fatigue and may end in suicide. Amok often manifests without warning, although some incidents are precipitated by a period of intense anxiety or hostility. *Koro/jinjin/bemar/suk/yeong/suo-yang* in Southeast Asia, south China, and India, is an acute panic or anxiety reaction involving fear of genital retraction (men fear their penis will withdraw into the abdomen; women fear withdrawal of their breasts, labia, or vulva). It is thought to be fatal.

- **Latin America.** In this area, *susto/espanto* (fright) has a diverse set of chronic complaints that are attributed to soul loss due to a severe, often supernatural, fright. Symptoms include agitation, anorexia, insomnia, fever, diarrhea, mental confusion, apathy, depression, and introversion. Among indigenous peoples in North America, the Inuit who live in the Arctic Circle area of North America and Asia can suffer from *pibloktoq* (arctic hysteria) which is characterized by fatigue, depression, or confusion followed by disruptive behavior that includes stripping off clothing, frenzied running, rolling in snow, glossolalia (repetitive nonmeaningful speech), echolalia (involuntary repeating of the utterances of another—associated with autism), echopraxia (involuntary repeating of the movements of another—associated with schizophrenia, Tourette's syndrome, and other neurological disorders), property destruction, and coprophagia (eating feces). Most episodes last only minutes and are followed by loss of consciousness, amnesia, and complete recovery.

CONCLUSION

In this geographic tour of theories of disease causation throughout the world I have provided a broad outline of what is important about belief systems and healing traditions in each geographic area both in the past and in the present. I have also repeatedly made the important point that medicine cannot be divorced from other cultural beliefs and institutions. In particular, knowledge of religious belief and general philosophy of life is often critical to understanding local medical theory and practices, especially for lay health care seeking behavior. Religious beliefs and philosophies about how the world works have always profoundly affected what is possible in medical practice, as exemplified by medieval Europe's prohibition of human dissection and the assault on therapeutic abortion and stem cell research in the United States today. They have also affected the kind of treatment that patients are willing to accept.

Throughout history, wherever civilizations have developed, their medical traditions have been elaborated and have become dominant in the areas under their sway. Yet, these great medical traditions have always existed and continue to exist alongside the other major medical traditions that were and are their contemporaries. Moreover, these formal medical traditions have also coexisted with the many informal local medical, healing, and belief systems that we have discussed in this book. All of these systems continually interact and exchange theories and techniques for healing and have done so for centuries. Medical systems are not static entities; they change over time, often radically with new knowledge, because the drive to heal and to be healed is such an important part of human life. At times these different systems are at odds, at times they are complementary, and at times they are synergistic. What they all have in common, however, is their attempt to return health to the ill.

With the tremendous advances in literacy and the stunning changes in access to information due to the Internet and other information technologies that have occurred in the last 25 years, our world has shrunk considerably. With the migration of large numbers of people, many from former colonies to the West, the former stability of national cultures has also broken down and all parts of the world have become increasingly multicultural. Thus, we can expect to see even more interaction and exchange among the different medical systems of the world as well as misunderstandings and misinterpretations between healers and patients like that so eloquently described by Anne Fadiman (1998) in *The Spirit Catches You and You Fall Down*, which chronicles the tragic story of misunderstandings surrounding the care of a Hmong child in the United States whose biomedical diagnosis of epilepsy conflicted with the family and community diagnosis of soul loss. The persistent importance of supernatural disease causation—both in the ethnographic past and in the present—throughout the world's many different cultures reflects a human need to try to explain that which is not understood. As physician-anthropologist Cecil Helman notes: "unpleasant, disembodied and 'non-self' emotions and feelings—those invaders of body and soul—are really the modern descendants of ancient devils, ghosts, dybbuks, and ancestral spirits—and all of the other invisible inhabitants of a parallel and mystical world" (Helman 2004:107).

In the final chapter, we explore the issue of cultural competence and what healers and patients need to understand about each other in order to navigate the sometimes vast differences in their explanatory models of disease and healing.

Notes

[1] I use the term *ethnographic past* for the time period portrayed in most of the classic ethnographies that are about groups whose ways of life were relatively untouched by modernization and who were studied well before globalization. The societies portrayed in these studies were the traditional subjects of anthropological inquiry. They were sought out for their difference and remoteness from Western society. Although no culture was ever truly isolated from at least some form of contact with other cultures, the degree of isolation was far greater than today.

[2] This older approach at cross-cultural understanding has been replaced today by multisited studies that use the same methodology and address the same research questions. The Human Relations Area Files at Yale University maintain a collection of thousands of full text sources on almost 400 cultures worldwide that can be accessed for information about specific societies or for cross-cultural research (http://www.yale.edu/hraf/index.html).

[3] Murdock instructed his staff not to code for this variable because of its seeming obviousness, which he later regretted. Thus, while violence and aggression in these societies are probably universal, this category was dropped from his study.

[4] Sorcery techniques included contagious magic, exuvial magic, imitative magic, object intrusion, presumptive poison, spirit possession, soul theft, and verbal spells.

[5] Murdock's witchcraft techniques included evil eye and "other." Although Murdock included evil eye under witchcraft, today it is considered as different from witchcraft because it is usually imparted accidentally by a person who has the affliction of being able to impart evil eye but not the control over it implied in witchcraft, which is a premeditated act.

[6] Taboo violations included those surrounding etiquette, food, ritual, sex, and sensory.

[7] "The word 'tzaddik' literally means 'righteous one.' The term refers to a completely righteous individual, and generally indicates that the person has spiritual or mystical power. A tzaddik is not necessarily a rebbe or a rabbi, but the rebbe of a Chasidic community is considered to be a tzaddik." http://www.jewfaq.org/rabbi.htm#Tzaddik (accessed 4/30/06).

[8] Traditionally the five major world religions include Judaism, Christianity, Islam, Hinduism, and Buddhism. By proportion of the world population, the major religious groups include: Christianity (33%), Islam (21%), Hinduism (13%), Buddhism (6%), traditional Chinese (6%), ethno religions (4%), other (4%), atheists (3%), and not religious (13%). http://www.religioustolerance.org/worldrel.htm (accessed 10/9/07).

[9] The Baha'i World Faith is also classified as an Abrahamic religion by some authorities. It developed in Iran in the mid-19th century and recognizes Adam, Krishna, Buddha, Jesus, Mohammed, The Bab (the Gate), who founded Baha'i and a later manifestation of The Bab, Baha'u'llah (the Glory of God), as Prophets through whom the word of God has been imparted to humans. The teachings of Baha'u'llah include world peace, democracy, civil rights, equal rights for women, and the acceptance of scientific discoveries, and were decades ahead of his time. http://www.religioustolerance.org/bahai.htm (accessed 9/17/07).

[10] Moses was the author of the first five books of the Torah/Old Testament and receiver of the Ten Commandments.

[11] The Church of Christ, Scientist Web site: http://www.tfccs.com/scienceandhealth/index.jhtml (accessed 2/26/06).

[12] For ease of differentiation and clarity, I use the term "spiritualism" for sects that developed from an explicitly Christian base that incorporates contact with the spirit world. I use the term "spiritism" for other traditions that incorporate contact with the spirit world that originated in other religious traditions.

[13] National Spiritualist Association of Churches website http://www.nsac.org/spiritualism/index.htm#SPIRITUAL%20HEALING (accessed 2/26/06).

[14] See Baer 2001 and 2004 and Gevitz 1988 for more detailed information.

[15] "Approximately 65% of all osteopathic physicians practice in primary care areas such as pediatrics, family practice, obstetrics/gynecology and internal medicine." American Osteopathic Association website http://www.osteopathic.org/index.cfm (accessed 2/19/06).

[16] American Chiropractic Association website http://www.amerchiro.org/ (accessed 2/19/06).

[17] National Center for Complementary and Alternative Medicine website: http://nccam.nih.gov/health/homeopathy (accessed 2/19/06).

[18] Homeopathic Educational Services website: http://www.homeopathic.com/articles/intro/ten_top_questions.php (accessed 2/19/06).

[19] Coalition for Natural Health website: http://www.naturalhealth.org/tradnaturo/history2.html#erop (accessed 2/26/06).

[20] Naturowatch website: http://www.naturowatch.org/licensure/laws.shtml and Natural Healers website, http://www.naturalhealers.com/qa/naturopathy.html#q1 (accessed 2/26/06).

[21] Kate Nolan, *The Arizona Republic*, April 11, 2005, 12:00 a.m., "Naturopaths to Get own Trade Publication" http://www.azcentral.com/community/scottsdale/articles/0411sr-journal11Z8.html.

[22] Native peoples of North and South America are thought to be descendants of indigenous groups from Siberia that migrated first to North America about 15,000 years ago via the Bering Strait land bridge and then to Central and South America. In the United States, indigenous peoples are known as Native Americans; in Canada as First Nations, although they often prefer to use their individual tribal names or, simply Columbus's misnomer, Indians.

[23] Australian aborigines are thought to have migrated from Southeast Asia to northern Australia some 40,000–50,000 years BCE. They appear not to be related to any known Asian group or to the Melanesian and Polynesian peoples geographically closest to them and were an isolated population for much of their time in Australia.

[24] For example, Olorum is associated with Jesus Christ or the dove of the Holy Spirit, Babalu-Aye (associated with diseases) with St. Lazarus, Obatala (father of the orisha) with Our Lady of Mercy, and Chango (ruler of lightning and thunder) with St. Barbara.

[25] Dahomey was a kingdom in Africa (now the nation of Benin). It was founded in the 17th century and survived until the late 19th century, when it was conquered by France. It was one of West Africa's principal slave states and was extremely unpopular with neighboring groups, especially the Yoruba, who were taken into slavery in large numbers.

[26] According to ethnobotanist, Wade Davis (1988), the drug is tetrodotoxin (a chemical found in the toxic puffer fish). If administered correctly, tetrodotoxin does not kill, but induces a coma that seems like death and lasts for about three days after which the person either dies or comes out of the coma. Administration of a different drug, datura, after the person comes out of the coma is what maintains the zombified state.

[27] The popular NBC sitcom ran from 1965–1970 and followed the adventures of Jeannie, a genie accidentally freed by an astronaut who finds her in a bottle, who grants her new master wishes that inevitably resolve in a well-meaning but comically unforeseen manner.

[28] http://muttaqun.com/jinn.html (accessed 9/17/07).

[29] The Moghul Empire dominated most of the Indian subcontinent during the 16th and 17th centuries, establishing Islam (first brought by Arab invaders in the 12th century) in India.

[30] Moxibustion is a therapy that uses *moxa* (mugwort plant) in fluff or stick form to warm (by burning it) an acupuncture point or area of the body in order to stimulate the circulation of the blood and/or qi. It can be used alone or with acupuncture needles.

[31] *The I Ching on the Net* website includes examples of readings from the hexagrams and associated texts, http://pacificcoast.net/~wh/Index.html (accessed 9/17/07).

[32] There are hundreds of gods and goddesses as well as saints, immortals, and demigods.

[33] Chinese astrology uses the Chinese agricultural calendar and its own Zodiac (12-year cycle of animals), the five elements of Chinese thought, calendar cycles based on astronomy, and ancient Chinese religion.

[34] Feng shui is the ancient Chinese practice of placement and arrangement of space to achieve harmony with the environment.

[35] Most worship involves bowing towards an altar, with a stick of incense, and may be done at home, in a temple, or outdoors, by an ordinary person or a professional. The altar can have any number of deities or ancestral tablets.

[36] Ch'ondogyo is a relatively new and increasingly important religion in Korea. It is a synthesis of Confucian, Buddhist, shamanistic, Taoist, and Catholic influences that grew out of the 19th century nationalistic Tonghak Movement. Its teachings include the essential equality of all human beings, each of whom must be treated with respect; that God exists in every person; and that self-perfection is the route to salvation. This religious movement was an important factor in the revolt against the royal government in 1894 that contributed to the development of democracy in Korea.

[37] Like China, Korea has a host of spirits that include the millions of gods and goddesses (from the "generals" who rule heaven to local gods of households and villages); nature spirits who inhabit stones, caves, etc.; mischievous goblins; and ghosts of dead people who met violent or tragic ends. All are thought to be able to influence the fortunes of living people.

[38] http://www.thai-massage.org/history.html, and http://www.taomountain.org/thai-medicine/thai-massage.html (both accessed 12/4/06).

Chapter 5

The Healing Lessons
of Ethnomedicine

I began this book by asking a question—what is ethnomedicine? I will end by asking three more questions. What do ethnomedicines, including biomedicine, tell us about the nature of disease and illness, curing and healing? What do the ethnomedicine lessons mean for cultural competence in biomedical care? What is the future of ethnomedicines in our globalized world?

WHAT DO ETHNOMEDICINES TELL US?

The comparative study of ethnomedicines provides a foundation for understanding the range of ethnomedical theory and practice that can help us to understand why healing can and does occur within all ethnomedical systems. In this book I have aimed to trace the broad similarities between ethnomedicines rather than focus on their particular differences. This section highlights the six major lessons we learned from looking systematically at ethnomedicines and then explains how these insights might be used by health practitioners to facilitate culturally appropriate health care in our international pluralistic health care system.

Lesson 1. Ethnomedicine is embedded in a cultural and environmental context. The historical and geographical tour of ethnomedicines we have taken in this book clearly shows us that all ethnomedical systems develop within a specific cultural, environmental, and historical context and that they reflect that culture and, in particular, the religious and philosophical beliefs about the place of human beings in the world and their relationship to the physical, social, spiritual, and supernatural environments. In fact, ethnomedical systems are so fully embedded in culture that they are difficult to understand without also understanding something about the parent culture. For example, TCM is baffling until one understands something about Tao, Buddhism, yin/yang, qi, and the underlying principle that illness is thought to be a result of imbalance or blockage of the normal flow of the life force. Similarly, biomedicine would seem bizarre to people who did not have an understanding of science and the reductionist model of disease that allows medicine to view the body as a machine that can be fixed by a physician. The biomedical clinical encounter would be positively alien to people who do not view the human body as something separate and detached from the mind, from social relations, and from nature. Biomedical physicians treat a decontextualized and often dehumanized individual physical body, sometimes even a part of a body (the heart, the leg, etc.). In this, biomedicine is unique among the ethnomedicines we have encountered in our exploration. Of course, many biomedical practitioners also recognize how this broader set of connections and contexts influence the health of their patients, but they have no vehicle within the biomedical system to address them.[1] Virtually all other ethnomedicines view a person holistically as a mind/body that is linked to the social, the political, the spiritual, the supernatural, and to nature, and they understand illness to be a disruption in the balance that must be maintained among all of these spheres.

Lesson 2. Ethnomedical systems change over time. Our tour has also shown us that ethnomedical systems are not static, closed systems. They have all benefited from interaction with other medical systems and have incorporated new treatments and medicines from systems that developed in other lands. There has been much interaction, exchange, and borrowing from one system to another throughout history. The pace of this exchange increased greatly after the Renaissance due to exploration and colonization, and it has increased again, astronomically so, over the past two decades due to globalization and the introduction of the new information technologies worldwide, but the interactive process is the same. Healers have always been interested in finding better ways to treat their patients, and patients have actively sought alternative means of healing. Thus, while the broad outlines of medical systems in different geographical areas tend to persist over time, the particular practices change through the processes of indigenous innovation and the borrowing and adapting of therapies and theories from other systems. The evolution of Unani medicine from Greek medicine is one example. The sculpting of Chinese medicine in Thailand and Korea to include native therapies and indigenous herbals while embracing TCM's underlying theory of disease causation is another. The emergence of CAM in the West and resulting pluralistic medical systems is a third example.

Lesson 3. Different ethnomedicines are hegemonic in different times and places. Greek medicine was the hegemonic system of Greece, the Roman Empire, and Europe for hundreds of years. Traditional Chinese medicine was hegemonic in East and Southeast Asia and Ayurvedic medicine dominated in West Asia for thousands of years. These great medical traditions became dominant in their regions through diffusion, imperialism, colonialism, and military and economic control. For the last five centuries the West has been the hegemonic political economic system in the world. Since the end of World War II, biomedicine has become the dominant global medical system, resulting in the institutionalization of its emphasis on tertiary, curative care at the apex of most medical systems. Biomedical prominence channels funding toward hospital-based medicine, draining funds for primary health care and prevention in the less-developed countries, with notable exceptions such as Cuba and the fleeting emphasis on Primary Health Care by WHO in the 1970s. Prevention has primarily been left to public health efforts through WHO and various other multilateral, unilateral, and national funders and increasingly through nongovernmental organizations (NGOs) that have fewer explicitly political motives than the government-based funders. We have also discussed the increasing resistance to the dominance of the biomedical model and an ever more persistent pressure among Western populations to broaden the scope of healing strategies in the West to include and legitimize (i.e., have health insurance cover) CAMs.

Lesson 4. The interdependence of mind and body and the social causes of illness are central to all ethnomedicines except biomedicine. On our tour of different ethnomedicines, biomedicine stands out as the only one that separates the mental from the physical. The fallout of this mind/body dualism, the legacy of Descartes, is a tendency to focus on disease rather than health. John Macdonald makes the important point that biomedicine exhibits "sometimes grotesque imbalances in health systems with institutions of care concerning themselves principally with disease and not with health" (Macdonald 2005:79). He draws attention to the fact that biomedicine still tends to decontextualize health and disease despite the "growing evidence of the centrality of context to many conditions of health and illness" (Macdonald 2005:79). Health and illness are the product of the person and his/her interaction with the environment writ large (i.e., built and natural environments, social, political-economic, spiritual and supernatural). The World Health Organization's report on the social determinants of health (Wilkinson and Marmot 2003) and the recent focus on researching and eliminating health disparities in the United States

(CDC 2007) speak to the need to expand understanding of health and disease from a focus on the decontextualized, physical body and its biological and molecular processes to a focus on the mind/body and the broader environment in which people live. It is now undeniable that "many of the most vexing and enduring health problems . . . are etiologically tied to a complex web of political, cultural, and economic conditions" (Stokols 2000:5) that exert a negative effect on health. It is also important to remember that the reverse is also true—positive social, political, cultural, and economic environments foster positive health outcomes and mediate response to misfortune. Macdonald makes an impassioned plea for biomedicine to recognize a life force, by which he means that innate ability of the human body and psyche to be self-healing. Biomedicine must acknowledge that all ethnomedicines simply facilitate or remove obstacles to this natural tendency of the body to heal itself. In thinking about illness and the efficacy of ethnomedicines, we must remember the 80% Rule that four out of five people who seek medical care get better regardless of their treatment actions. It is the natural tendency of the body to heal itself that is augmented by ethnomedicines.

Lesson 5. Ethnomedicines recognize four major domains of disease causation and three theories that explain the disease process. In chapter 3 we reviewed many different things that people think can cause disease. These can be categorized into four broad domains: the individual body (e.g., genetic makeup, personality, lifestyle, emotions, nutrition, age, etc.); the natural world (e.g., environment, climate, toxins, natural disasters, flora and fauna, water, etc.); the social and economic world (e.g., poverty, warfare, violence, social support, etc.); and the supernatural and spiritual world (e.g., God, gods, sin, witchcraft, sorcery, soul loss, etc.). In addition there are three broad theories that explain the process of illness within these domains: imbalance (humors, hot/cold, cholesterol, energy, humans with nature, etc.); natural pathogenic processes (infection, degeneration, etc.); and punishment for offenses committed wittingly or not (against nature, other people, God, spirits, etc., or karma). The four domains of causation and the three theories of disease process are not necessarily mutually exclusive within or across different ethnomedicines, although we noted that societies have a tendency toward natural vs. supernatural explanations and impersonal vs. personalistic explanations.

For example, Ayurvedic medicine relies on the theory of balance and a tendency toward naturalistic explanations of illness. It also tends to treat at the individual and social levels, but within a holistic framework that can accommodate the natural and the supernatural as well. Imbalance can be manifested within the body itself as well as between the person and his/her social, natural, and supernatural spheres. Navajo medicine, by contrast, relies a great deal on supernatural explanations of illness and a theory of imbalance of the individual with nature and the supernatural. It tends to treat at the supernatural level. At the other extreme, biomedicine tends toward naturalistic explanations and theories of pathogenic processes and treatment occurs within the domain of the individual body. Biomedicine rejects the supernatural as cause of disease, but many Western patients still invoke religion to heal disease. Indeed, many biomedical health practitioners simultaneously maintain scientific theories as well as beliefs about spirituality. In sum, there is wide variation in ethnomedicines regarding these dimensions of causation and foci of treatment. Practitioners of any ethnomedicine might increase their effectiveness by being aware of the range of illness and healing beliefs they may encounter in caring for patients, especially those from of other cultural backgrounds.

One of the things driving interest in CAM in the West is the ability of other ethnomedicines to address domains that remain outside of the biomedical purview.[2] Westerners seem to be seeking a reintegration of mind and body and to want their health care system to address relationships to the social, natural, and supernatural worlds. Perhaps Westerners are seeking restoration of harmony and balance in all four domains of their lives. Macdonald suggests that health needs to be reframed as a positive interaction with the environment, a constant adaptation to maintain homeostasis (balance between competing influences), not with just the physical environment, but also with "the social, cultural, economic and psychological and spiritual worlds of people" (Macdonald 2005:90). Health, then, should be reframed as a balance among all of these domains of human life.

A case in point is global warming. It is impossible to deny the truth of global warming any longer or the fact that its cause is due to industrialization and automobiles, the world's militaries' use of oil (the largest single polluter), deforestation (associated with overpopulation, poverty, unsustainable farming, and logging), and combustion for cooking and heating (Donohoe 2007). The West is primarily responsible for global warming, but the South will be affected the most by it. One of the results of global warming is the melting of the polar ice caps and glaciers, raising global sea levels and increasing coastal erosion and flooding. Another is the augmentation of the effects of extreme weather patterns like El Niño. The third major result is depletion of the ozone layer and increasing air pollution. All of these outcomes of global warming will be associated with significant morbidity and mortality (Donohoe 2007). Expanding the notion of health to include balance with nature, the social and cultural, the economic, and the spiritual[3] worlds of people could assist in the struggle for a better world by providing a philosophical and moral basis for addressing environmental problems, cultural destruction, violence, poverty, and inequality as issues of health and human rights. Balance and equity promote health.

Lesson 6. The purpose of ethnomedicines is both to heal and to cure. For all humans, illness is one of the many misfortunes that are part of life. The purpose of ethnomedical systems is to alleviate the suffering of patients who are ill. To do so, all ethnomedical systems have developed strategies to treat illness that include diagnosis, treatment, and cure or amelioration. In addition they outline a path for both prevention of illness and for restoration of health (treatment plan), and sometimes they provide the patient with an idea of his/her chances of recovery (prognosis). Finally, they often answer the big questions of why and how the patient came to bear the misfortune of illness. This bigger question is not part of official biomedicine, which stops at the scientific explanation. All patients, however, search for a larger meaning and an explanation that interprets misfortune, especially serious illness, in the context of our cosmological place in the world. Patients search for both healing (restoration of physical, mental, emotional, social, and spiritual health) and curing (removal or correction of organic pathology). Biomedicine fails in this larger contextualization because its theory of disease causation is too narrow to accommodate such cosmological and existential questions about human existence. Thus, Western patients are turning increasingly to CAM, and biomedicine is gradually becoming one of the many ethnomedicines from which people can choose.

WHAT DO THE ETHNOMEDICINE LESSONS MEAN FOR CULTURAL COMPETENCE IN BIOMEDICAL CARE?

It is impossible for any health practitioner to learn all of the particularities of all ethnomedicines in the world, but it is possible to have an understanding of major theories of disease causation that underlie ethnomedicines and knowledge of their geographical distribution. It is also possible to be mindful that the explanatory models of disease/illness are likely to differ between patients and providers. Patients have their own ideas about what caused their health problem based on their individual and cultural understanding of health and illness. In biomedical care, as Kleinman (1980) reminds us, it is always important to compare the physician's and the patient's explanatory models of causation to determine similarities and differences between them and to come to an understanding about treatment that can accommodate both perspectives. The goal for any health care practitioner and his/her patient is restoration of health. Respectful consideration of the patient's view and careful explanation of the practitioner's view go a long way to improve understanding that will, in turn, foster greater adherence to treatment regimens. Practitioner and patient do not necessarily have to agree about causation, but they must find a common ground for treatment that meets both of their needs. This may mean that biomedical practitioners need to encourage complementary and alternative treatment strategies favored by patients along with biomedical strategies; because the treatment must fit both the patient's and the practitioner's needs to be successful. Nonadherence to treatment regimens may indicate a mismatch in theories of disease/illness causation rather than a rejection of the desire to get well.

The hallmark of a multicultural approach to health care is acknowledging, valuing, and respecting all cultures', religions', and ethnicities' theories of disease causation, something that is alien to the West's belief in science and the resulting ethnocentric belief that Western medical traditions are superior to those of the rest of the world. The crux of cultural competence for biomedicine is how to reconcile its own belief that the scientific method supersedes all other theoretical paradigms of medical explanation with the inevitable realization that not everyone in the world believes this, that other systems "work," and yet patients from different traditions and those from the West who seek alternative care still seek biomedical care. Patients are using a pluralistic system, and biomedicine would benefit by accommodating this reality.

A second lesson for culturally competent health care from the study of ethnomedicines is that the social context of decision making regarding treatment for many societies is not individual-based as it is in the West. Biomedicine generally recognizes only the individual as the center of care and decision-making power except in cases where individuals are not legally competent to decide for themselves (e.g., children and the mentally incompetent). The West is unusual in its allocation of decision-making authority to the individual patient. Many cultures have a more collectivistic approach to social organization and to therapy management and decision making about patient care. In some societies, for example, the eldest relatives in the extended family make decisions about health care. In others, the husband or male head of household decides. Whatever the constellation of decision-making power, it behooves the biomedical practitioner to discover it and utilize it in case management, because who makes decisions about treatment affects patient care.

A third lesson from ethnomedicines is that there are significant differences between Western and non-Western cultures in how they view the relationship of humans to the environment as well as the degree of agency human beings have in their lives. The West, for example, favors mastery over nature rather than harmony with it and personal control of behavior to determine one's own destiny, rather than the idea that fate or destiny might be preordained. It favors science over religion and objective knowledge over intuitive, subjective understandings. The West values an orientation toward time and money rather than social relations to organize society. It privileges young adults over elders and children; directness and openness in dealings with others over indirectness and ritualization of interaction; informality over formality; and future orientation over veneration of the past (Coe n.d.). The West, essentially, privileges the rational over the metaphysical, the new/young over the traditional/old, and the accumulation of things over social capital. This reverses the norms on which social organization was based for much of the history of human existence and still exist in many contemporary societies today.

The final lesson from the study of ethnomedicines is that multiple use of different medical systems is already common among patients in Western, perhaps all, societies and should be considered normative. There have been endless discussions about why this is the case, most of which point to the failure of biomedicine to be holistic—to treat the patient in social, economic, and spiritual/cosmological context—or to be successful in treatment of chronic or otherwise nonresponsive health conditions. I suspect that both reasons apply. The West is facing a crisis of belief in its medical system. Patients want something it is not capable of delivering, hence the ever more pluralistic nature of health-care-seeking behavior. In the end, patients will seek the care that they need based on their evaluation of the merits of the practitioners and therapies offered and their understanding of their health problem. With the emergence of evidence-based medicine, the epitome of rational scientific medicine notwithstanding, many patients are voting with their feet and their wallets to use other healing traditions that consider matters not addressed by biomedicine. It is unfortunate that epistemological wars are created over the science/religion, objective/subjective, rational/magical debates that accompany debates over biomedicine and CAM. Humans have the capacity to simultaneously hold and reconcile competing ideas about the nature of the universe. It is not at all surprising to find religious biomedical physicians (rather than atheists) or empirical herbalists who subscribe to the mystical (rather than natural) properties of their cures. The mystical and the empirical are intertwined in the human understanding of the world. Like yin and yang, they are mutually necessary and inseparable.

Of course it is essential to have translation services for non-English-speaking patients in U.S. health care facilities. Nevertheless, it is also important for biomedical practitioners serving patients from different cultural groups to familiarize themselves with the major theories of disease causation in the particular cultural group with which they work. They must furthermore have a basic understanding of the composition of the normative therapy management group and those responsible for decision making about treatment and recognize that there is variation in both knowledge of and belief in traditional healing systems within cultural groups, which is largely based on education and acculturation level. A combination of active listening to patients' explanatory models, respect for beliefs that are not scientific, and suspension of judgmental, condescending attitudes when encountering different explanatory models of disease causation will go a long way toward instilling trust in patients. Faith and trust are essential components of healing for both patients and healers. They are essential for successful outcomes.

In the end, "cultural competency involves the understanding that increased knowledge of the role culture plays in shaping our attitudes, values, beliefs, and behaviors will lead to more culturally appropriate care, better health outcomes, and reduced health disparities" (Coe n.d.). Rather than a clash between biomedicine and CAM, there should be collaboration.

THE FUTURE OF ETHNOMEDICINES

Ethnomedical systems persist because they perform the valuable function of restoring members of society to healthy function, ameliorate chronic problems, and/or bring patients to resolution, acceptance, and understanding of that which does not respond to treatment. They are perceived to be effective by both their practitioners and patients. That nonbiomedical systems are effective can no longer be denied. Some therapies have been proven to be effective in scientific studies (e.g., herbal remedies, acupuncture). Others have not. This is also true of biomedical treatments, however, many of which have not been subjected to rigorous efficacy testing either. The interest in explaining successful CAM therapies in biomedical terms attests to the West's increasing acceptance of the idea that other ethnomedicines can be effective and understood within the scientific framework.

Recent scientific research has expanded our understanding of the human body, the brain, and the psycho-neuro-immune pathways that link mind and body and allow the social, economic, and political (both negative and positive experiences) to become embodied (Krieger 2001, 2005, Singer and Clair 2003, Wilce 2003). As scientific researchers note, "The connections between the neoroendocrine system and immune system provide a finely tuned regulatory system required for health. *Disturbances* at any level of the HPA axis or glucocorticoid action *lead to an imbalance of this system* [emphasis added] and enhanced susceptibility to infection and inflammatory or autoimmune disease" (Webster et al. 2002:128). Reading this, we might hope that biomedicine could return to its roots in humoral medicine where body, mind, and spirit were thought of as the intertwined whole that constitutes a person. The radical approach taken by biomedicine in treating only the physical body has been unique in the history of medical systems. Perhaps the time has come for biomedicine to reinvent itself and take notice of the fact that its clients are demanding a more holistic perspective from their healers. Indeed, we may actually be living through a paradigm shift in the West during which our appreciation for both the efficacy of biomedicine and for the holistic patient-centeredness of CAM will result in a new way of understanding and doing prevention and curing within an integrated health care system (Bates 2000).

One thing is clear, there seems to be an acutely felt need in the West to find balance and tranquility in our increasingly complex and unbalanced world, but even if we have all the ethnomedical systems in the world to choose from in our quest for health, curing, restoration, and renewal, it is all for naught if we cannot avail ourselves of these services. As Baer reminds us "The creation of an authentically holistic and pluralistic medical system ultimately will have to be coupled with the demand for a universal health care system, one that incorporates alternative therapies and that treats health care as a right rather than a privilege" (2001:189).

Notes

[1] Many biomedical practitioners attempt to change the system from within and from without by incorporating CAM and social workers into the system, but addressing treatment and prevention issues that lie outside of the individual body must often be done on their own time outside of the institution through activities such as political pressure to reduce health disparities, personal spiritual involvement, participation in conservation movements, etc.

[2] Of course, CAM is also an industry driven by the same market economy as biomedicine, but greater consumer interest in CAM allows the industry to flourish and expand.

[3] The spiritual domain refers not only to the God, gods, Buddha, Nirvana, etc. of the major world religions but also to the many smaller gods and spirits believed to inhabit the world; to ghosts; to the metaphysical, cosmological and existential theories of being; to the awe of the natural environment; all of which make up the variety of spiritual and metaphysical experiences of human beings.

References

Ackernecht, Erwin. 1982. *A Short History of Medicine*. Baltimore: Johns Hopkins University Press.

American Medical Association. 1999. Child Abuse and Neglect. http://www.medem.com/search/article_display.cfm?path=n:&mstr=/ZZZBRKN PVAC.html&soc=AMA&srch_typ=NAV_SERCH (accessed 1/30/05).

American Psychiatric Association. 1994. *Diagnostic and Statistical Manual of Mental Disorders,* Fourth Edition. Washington, DC: American Psychiatric Association.

Armelagos, George J., Alan H. Goodman, and Kenneth Jacobs. 1991. "The Origins of Agriculture: Population Growth During a Period of Declining Health." In *Cultural Change and Population Growth: An Evolutionary Perspective*, Warren M. Hern (ed.). *Population and Environment* 13(1): 9–22.

Arvigo, Rosita. 1994. *Sastun: My Apprenticeship with a Maya Healer*. San Francisco, CA: HarperCollins.

Baasher, Taha. 1983. "The Eastern Mediterranean Region." In *Traditional Medicine and Health Care Coverage*, Robert H. Bannerman, John Burton, and Ch'en Wen-Chieh (eds.), pp. 253–262. Geneva: World Health Organization.

Baer, Hans. 2001. *Biomedicine and Alternative Healing Systems in America: Issues of Class, Race, Ethnicity, and Gender*. Madison: University of Wisconsin Press.

Baer, Hans. 2004. *Toward an Integrative Medicine: Merging Alternative Therapies with Biomedicine*. Walnut Creek, CA: AltaMira Press.

Baer, Hans A., Merrill Singer, and Ida Susser. 2003. *Medical Anthropology and the World System: A Critical Perspective*, 2nd Edition. Westport CT: Praeger.

Balick, Michael J. and Paul Alan Cox. 1996. *Plants, People, and Culture: The Science of Ethnobotany*. New York: Scientific American Library.

Balikci, Asen. 1967. "Shamanistic Behavior among the Netsilik Eskimos." In *Magic, Witchcraft, and Curing*, John Middleton (ed.), pp. 191–209. Austin: University of Texas Press.

Bannerman, Robert H., John Burton, and Ch'en Wen-Chieh (Eds.). 1983. *Traditional Medicine and Health Care Coverage*. Geneva: World Health Organization.

Basch, Paul F. 1999. *Textbook of International Health*. New York: Oxford University Press.

Bates, Don G. 2000. "Why Not Call Modern Medicine 'Alternative'"? *Perspectives in Biology and Medicine* 43(4): 502–518.

Beinfield, Harriet and Efrem Korngold. 1995. "Chinese Traditional Medicine: An Introductory Overivew." *Alternative Therapies* 1(1): 44–52.

Berman, Brian M., James P. Swyers, Susan M. Hartnoll, Betsy B. Singh, and Barker Bausell. 2000. "The Public Debate over Alternative Medicine: The Importance of Finding a Middle Ground." *Alternative Therapies* 6(1): 98–101.

Bernard, H. Russell. 2005. *Research Methods in Anthropology*, Fourth Edition. Lanham, MD: AltaMira.

Blaxter, Mildred. 2004. *Health*. Cambridge, UK: Polity Press.

Bodley, John. 2000. *Anthropology and Contemporary Human Problems*. New York: McGraw-Hill.

Boserup, Esther. 1981. *Population and Technological Change: A Study of Long-term Trends*. Chicago: University of Chicago Press.

Brewer, Harry. 2004. "Historical Perspectives on Health: Early Arabic Medicine." *Journal of the Royal Society for the Promotion of Health* 124(4): 184–187.

Brodwin, Paul E. 1992. "Guardian Angels and Dirty Spirits: The Moral Basis of Healing Power in Rural Haiti." In *Anthropological Approaches to the Study of Ethnomedicine*, Mark Nichter (ed.). pp. 57–74. Amsterdam: Gordon and Breach Science Publishers.

Brun, Viggo. 2003. "Traditional Thai Medicine." In *Medicine across Cultures*, H. Selin (ed.), pp. 115–132. Dordrecht, Netherlands: Kluwer Academic (Springer).

Buckley, Thomas and Alma Gottlieb (Eds.). 1988. *Blood Magic: The Anthropology of Menstruation*. Berkeley: University of California Press.

Caldwell, John C., Salley Findley, Pat Caldwell, Gigi Santow, Wendy Cosford, Jennifer Braid and Daphne Broers-Freeman (Eds.). 1990. *What We Know about the Health Transition: The Cultural, Social, and Behavioral Determinants of Health*, 2 volumes. Canberra, Australia: Australian National University Press.

CDC (Centers for Disease Control). 2007. *Eliminating Health Disparities*, http://www.cdc.gov/omh/About/disparities.htmboth (accessed 2/19/07).

Chang, Healani K. 2001. "Hawaiian Health Practitioners in Contemporary Society." *Pacific Health Dialog* 8(2): 260–273.

Coe, Kathryn. n.d. Multicultural Health Beliefs, Competency, and Ethics: The Importance of Culture and Cultural Competency in Patient Care. PowerPoint presentation. Arizona Cancer Center, Mel and Enid Zuckerman College of Public Health, Tucson, AZ.

Cohen, Ken ("Bear Hawk"). 1998. "Native American Medicine." *Alternative Therapies* 4(6): 45–56.

Coker, Ann L., Keith E. Davis, Ileana Arias, Sujata Desai, Maureen Sanderson, Heather M. Brandt, Paige H. Smith. 2002. "Physical and Mental Health Effects of Intimate Partner Violence for Men and Women." *American Journal of Preventive Medicine* 23(4): 260–268.

Davis, Wade. 1988. *Passage of Darkness: The Ethnobiology of the Haitian Zombie*. Chapel Hill: University of North Carolina Press.

DeNavas-Walt, Carmen, Bernadette D. Proctor, and Cheryl Hill Lee. 2005. "Income, Poverty, and Health Insurance Coverage in the United States: 2004." *U.S. Census Bureau, Current Population Reports, P60-229*. Washington, DC: U.S. Government Printing Office.

Diamond, Jared. 1999. *Guns, Germs, and Steel: The Fates of Human Societies*. New York: S. S. Norton.

Dobkin de Rios, Marlene. 1996. *Hallucinogens: Cross-Cultural Perspectives*. Long Grove, IL: Waveland Press.

Donohoe, Martin. 2007. "Global Warming: A Public Health Crisis Demanding Immediate Attention - Part 1." Medscape Public Health & Prevention. Posted 1/16/2007. http://www.medscape.com/viewarticle/548985.

Dossey, Larry. 1998. "The Evil Eye." *Alternative Therapies* 4(1): 9–18.

Dundes, Alan (Ed.). 1981. *The Evil Eye: A Folklore Casebook*. New York: Garland.

Editorial. 2006. "Time for the Renaissance of Medicine in the Middle East." *The Lancet* 367(9515): 959.

Ehrlich, Paul and Anne Ehrlich. 1991 [1990]. *The Population Explosion*. New York: Simon and Schuster.

Eisenberg, David M., Roger B. Davis, Susan L. Ettner, Scott Appel, Sonja Wilkey, Maria Van Rompay, and Ronald C. Kessler. 1998. "Trends in Alternative Medicine Use in the United States 1990–1997: Results of a Follow-up National Survey." *Journal of the American Medical Association* 280:1569–1575.

Eisenberg, Leon. 1977. "Disease and Illness: Distinctions between Professional and Popular Ideas of Sickness." *Medicine and Psychiatry* 1:9–23.

Eliade, Mircea. 1989 [1951]. *Shamanism. Archaic Techniques of Ecstasy*. London: Arkana.

Engebretson, Joan. 1998. "A Heterodox Model of Healing." *Alternative Therapies* 4(2): 37–43.

Epel, Elissa S., Elizabeth H. Blackburn, Jue Lin, Firdaus S. Dhabhar, Nancy E. Adler, Jason D. Morrow, and Richard M. Cawthon. 2004, December 7. "Accelerated Telomere Shortening in Response to Life Stress." *Proceedings of the National Academy of Sciences (PNAS)* 101(49): 17312–17315.

Erickson, Pamela I. In Press. "Revenge, Bride Capture, and Gender Strategies for Survival among the Waorani." In, *Revenge in Amazonia*, Stephen J. Beckerman and Paul Valentine (eds.). Gainesville: University Press of Florida.

Ernst, Edzard. 2000. "Assessing the Evidence Base for CAM." In *Complementary and Alternative Medicine: Challenge and Change*, Merrijoy Kelner et al. (eds.), pp. 165–173. Amsterdam: Harwood Academic Publishers.

Fadiman, Anne. 1998. *The Spirit Catches You and You Fall Down*. New York: Farrar, Strauss, and Giroux.

Foster, George M. 1953. "Relations between Spanish and Spanish-American Folk Medicine." *Journal of American Folklore* 66:201–217.

Foster, George M. 1976. "Disease Etiologies in Non-Western Medical Systems." *American Anthropologist* 78(4): 773–783.

Foster, George M. 1983. "An Introduction to Ethnomedicine." In *Traditional Medicine and Health Care Coverage*, Robert H. Bannerman, John Burton, and Ch'en Wen-Chieh (eds.), pp. 17–24. Geneva: World Health Organization.

Foster, George M. and Barbara Gallatin Anderson. 1978. *Medical Anthropology*. New York: John Wiley & Sons.

Fox, Ellen. 1997. "Predominance of the Curative Model of Medical Care: A Residual Problem?" *Journal of the American Medical Association* 278:761–763.

Frazer, Sir James George. 1940 [1922]. *The Golden Bough: A Study in Magic and Religion*. Volume I, Abridged Edition. New York: The Macmillan Company.

Frenk, Julio José-Luis Bobadilla, Claudio Stern, Tomas Frejka, and Rafael Lozano. 1993. "Elements for a Theory of the Health Transition." In *Health and Social Changes in International Perspective*, Lincoln Chen, Arthur Kleinman and Norma C. Ware (eds.), pp. 25–49. Boston, MA: Department of Population and International Health, Harvard School of Public Health, Distributed by Harvard University Press.

Frierman, Steven. 1985. "Struggles for Control: The Social Roots of Health and Healing in Modern Africa." *African Studies Review* 28(2/3): 73–147.

Gevitz, Norman (Ed.). 1988. *Other Healers. Unorthodox Medicine in America*. Baltimore: The Johns Hopkins University Press.

Goldwater, Carmel. 1983. "Traditional Medicine in Latin America." In *Traditional Medicine and Health Care Coverage*, Robert H. Bannerman, John Burton, and Ch'en Wen-Chieh (eds.), pp. 37–49. Geneva: World Health Organization.

Good, Byron 1977. "The Heart of What's the Matter: The Semantics of Illness in Iran." *Culture, Psychiatry and Medicine* 1:25–58.

Good, Byron and Mary-Jo Delvecchio Good. 1981. The Meaning of Symptoms: A Cultural Hermeneutic Model for Clinical Practice. In *The Relevance of Social Science for Medicine*, Leon Eisenberg and Arthur Kleinman (eds.), pp. 165–196. Hingham, MA: D. Reidel.

Green, Arthur. 2003. *Judaism and Healing: A Mystical Seeker's Perspective*. Hebrew Union College-Jewish Institute of Religion, Kalasman Institute on Judaism and Health. Temple Chai of Phoenix Deutsch Family Shalom Center. http://www.huc.edu/kalsman/projects/mining/green.pdf

Green, Edward C. 1999. *Indigenous Theories of Contagious Disease*. Walnut Creek, CA: AltaMira Press.

Hahn, Robert A. 1983. "Biomedical Practice and Anthropological Theory: Frameworks and Directions." *Annual Review of Anthropology* 12:305–333.

Hall, Edward T. 1969. *The Hidden Dimension*. New York: Anchor Books.

Halliburton, Murphy. 2005. "'Just Some Spirits': The Erosion of Spirit Possession and the Rise of 'Tension' in South India." *Medical Anthropology* 24(2): 111–144.

Harrell, Jules, Sadkli Hall, and James Taliaferro. 2003. "Physiological Responses to Racism and Discrimination: An Assessment o the Evidence." *American Journal of Public Health* 93(2): 243–248.

Harner, Michael J. 1972. *The Jívaro. People of the Sacred Waterfalls*. Berkeley: University of California Press.

Healthy People. 2000. *Healthy People 2000 Final Review: National Health Promotion and Disease Prevention Objectives*. Washington, DC: U.S. Department of Health and Human Services.

Helman, Cecil. 2004 [1992]. *The Body of Frankenstein's Monster: Essays in Myth and Medicine*. New York: Paraview Special Editions.

Helman, Cecil G. 2000. *Culture, Health and Illness*. Fourth Edition. Oxford: Butterworth-Heinemann.

Heymann, David L., James Cin, and Jonathan M. Mann. 1990. A Global Overview of AIDS. In *Heterosexual Transmission of Aids*, Nancy J. Alexander, Henry L. Gabelnick, and Jeffrey M. Spieler (eds.), pp. 1–8. New York: Wiley-Liss.

Hill, Kim, A. Magdalena Hurtado, R. S. Walker. 2007. "High Adult Mortality among Hiwi Hunter-Gatherers: Implications for Human Evolution." *Journal of Human Evolution* 52:443–454.

Holliday, Ian. 2003. "Traditional Medicines in Modern Societies: An Exploration of Integrationist Options through East Asian Experience." *Journal of Medicine and Philosophy* 28(3): 373–389.

Hughes, Charles C. 1968. "Ethnomedicine." *International Encyclopedia of the Social Sciences* 10:87–93. New York: Free Press/Macmillan.

Hughes, Charles C. 1985. Culture Bound or Construct Bound? The Syndromes and DSM-III. In *The Culture-Bound Syndromes: Folk Illnesses of Psychiatric and Anthropological Interest*, Ronald C. Simons and Charles C. Hughes (eds.), pp. 3–24. Dordrecht: D. Reidel.

Huntington, Samuel Phillips. 1996. *The Clash of Civilizations and the Remaking of World Order*. New York: Simon & Schuster.

Hyder, Adnana Ali and Richsar H. Morrow. 2001. Disease Burden Measurement and Trends. In *International Public Health: Diseases, Programs, Systems, and Policies*, Michael H. Merson, Robert E. Black, and Anne J. Mills (eds.), pp. 1–52. Gaithersburg, MD: Aspen.

Ibrahim, Said A. 2003. "Achieving Health Equity an Incremental Journey." *American Journal of Public Health* 93(10): 1619–1621.

Jakobsen, Marete Demant. 1999. *Shamanism: Traditional and Contemporary Approaches to the Mastery of Spirits and Healing*. New York and Oxford: Berghahn.

Janes, Craig R. 1999. "The Health Transition, Global Modernity and the Crisis of Traditional Medicine: The Tibetan Case" *Social Science and Medicine* 48(12): 1803–1820.

Jankowiak, William (Ed.). 1995. *Romantic Passion: A Universal Experience?* New York: Columbia University Press.

Janzen, John. 1978. *The Quest for Therapy in Lower Zaire*. Berkeley: University of California Press.

Janzen, John M. 2002. *The Social Fabric of Health: An Introduction to Medical Anthropology*. New York: McGraw-Hill.

Jilek, Wolfgang G. 2001. Cultural Factors in Psychiatric Disorders. Paper presented at the 26th Congress of the World Federation for Mental Health, July 2001, http://mentalhealth.com/mag1/wolfgang.html (accessed 1/16/06).

Jonas, Wayne. 2000. "The Social Dynamics of Medical Pluralism." In *Complementary and Alternative Medicine: Challenge and Change*, Merrijoy Kelner, Beverly Wellman, Bernice Pescosolido, and Mike Saks (eds.), pp. xi–xv. Amsterdam: Harwood Academic Publishers.

Joralemon, Donald and Douglas Sharon. 1993. *Sorcery and Shamanism, Curanderos and Clients in Northern Peru*. Salt Lake City: University of Utah Press.

Karlsen, Saffron and James Y. Nazroo. 2002a. "Relation between Racial Discrimination, Social Class, and Health among Ethnic Minority Groups." *Research and Practice* 92(4): 624–631.

Karlsen, Saffron and James Y. Nazroo. 2002b. "Agency and Structure: The Impact of Ethnic Identity and Racism on the Health of Ethnic Minority People." *Sociology of Health and Illness* 24(1):1–20.

Kehoe, Alice Beck. 2000. *Shamans and Religion: An Exploration in Critical Thinking.* Long Grove, IL: Waveland Press.

Kelner, Merrijoy, Beverly Wellman, Bernice Pescosolido, and Mike Saks (Eds.). 2000. *Complementary and Alternative Medicine: Challenge and Change.* Amsterdam: Harwood Academic Publishers.

Kelner, Merrijoy and Beverly Wellman. 2000. "Introduction." In *Complementary and Alternative Medicine: Challenge and Change,* Merrijoy Kelner, Beverly Wellman, Bernice Pescosolido, and Mike Saks (eds.), pp. 1–24. Amsterdam: Harwood Academic Publishers.

Kleinman, Arthur. 1980. *Patients and Healers in the Context of Culture.* Berkeley: University of California Press.

Kleinman, Arthur, L. Eisenberg, and Byron Good. 1978. "Culture, Illness, and Care: Clinical Lessons from Anthropologic and Cross-cultural Research." *Annals of Internal Medicine* 88:251–258.

Kleinman, Arthur, Peter Kunstadter, E. Russell Alexander, James L. Gale (Eds.). 1975. *Medicine in Chinese Cultures.* Washington, DC: U. S. Department of Health, Education and Welfare.

Kluckhohn, Clyde and Dorothea Leighton. 1962. *The Navajo.* The American Museum of National History Library Revised Edition. New York: Anchor Books, Doubleday.

Koenig, Harold G., Ellen Idler, Stanislav Kasl, Judith C. Hays, Linda K. George, Marc Musick, David B. Larson, Terence R. Collins, and Herbert Benson. 1999. "Religion, Spirituality, and Medicine: A Rebuttal to Skeptics." *International Journal of Psychiatry and Medicine* 29:123–131.

Koumaré, Mamadou. 1983. "Traditional Medicine and Psychiatry in Africa." In *Traditional Medicine and Health Care Coverage,* Robert H. Bannerman, John Burton, and Ch'en Wen-Chieh (eds.), pp. 25–32. Geneva: World Health Organization.

Krieger, Nancy. 2001. "Theories for Social Epidemiology in the 21st Century: An Ecosocial Perspective." *International Journal of Epidemiology* 20(4): 668–677.

Krieger, Nancy. 2005. "Embodiment: A Conceptual Glossary for Epidemiology." *Journal of Epidemiology and Community Health* 59:350–355.

Kunitz, Stephen J. 1989. *Disease Change and the Role of Medicine: The Navajo Experience.* Berkeley: University of California Press.

Kun, Kuang An. 1983. "The Western Pacific Region." In *Traditional Medicine and Health Care Coverage,* Robert H. Bannerman, John Burton, and Ch'en Wen-Chieh (eds.), pp. 263–278. Geneva: World Health Organization.

Kunow, Marianna Appel. 2003. *Maya Medicine: Traditional Healing in Yucatán.* Albuquerque: University of New Mexico Press.

Kurup, P. N. V. 1983. "Ayurveda." In *Traditional Medicine and Health Care Coverage,* Robert H. Bannerman, John Burton, and Ch'en Wen-Chieh (eds.), pp. 50–60. Geneva: World Health Organization.

Lad, Vasant. 1995. "An Introduction to Ayurveda." *Alternative Therapies* 1(3): 57–63.

Laguerre, Michel. 1987. *Afro-Caribbean Folk Medicine*. South Hadley, MA: Bergin & Garvey.

Landy, David. 1977. "Medical Systems in Transcultural Perspective." In *Culture, Disease, and Healing: Studies in Medical Anthropology*, David Landy (ed.), pp. 129–132. New York: Macmillan.

Levy, Barry S. and Victor W. Sidel (Eds.). 2000. *War and Public Health*. Updated Edition. Washington, DC: American Public Health Association.

Lewis, Walter Hepworth and Memory P. F. Elvin-Lewis. 2003. *Medical Botany: Plants Affecting Human Health*. Hoboken, New Jersey: John Wiley & Sons.

Lock, Margaret and Nancy Scheper-Hughes. 1996. "A Critical-Interpretive Approach in Medical Anthropology: Rituals and Routines of Discipline and Dissent." In *Medical Anthropology: Contemporary Theory and Method*, Carolyn F. Sargent and Thomas M. Johnson (eds.), pp. 41–70. Westport, CT: Praeger.

Logan, Michael H. 1972. "Humoral Folk Medicine: A Potential Aid in Controlling Pellagra in Mexico." *Ethnomedizin* 4:397–410.

Logan, Michael H. 1973. "Humoral Medicine in Guatemala and Peasant Adoption of Modern Medicine." *Human Organization* 32(1): 385–395.

Lovallo, William R. 1997. *Stress and Health: Biological and Psychological Interactions*. Thousand Oaks, CA: Sage.

Macdonald, John J. 2005. *Environments for Health*. London: Earthscan.

Magner, Lois N. 2005. *A History of Medicine*. Second Edition. New York: Taylor & Francis.

Mandelbaum, David G. 1970. "The Social Relevance of Ritual Purity and Pollution, Society in India." *Continuity and Change*. Volume One, pp. 192–205. Berkeley: University of California Press.

McElroy, Ann and Patricia K. Townsend. 2004. *Medical Anthropology in Ecological Perspective*. Fourth Edition. Boulder, CO: Westview Press.

McGuire, Meredith. 1988. *Ritual Healing in Suburban America*. New Brunswick, NJ: Rutgers University Press.

McNeill, William H. 1976. *Plagues and Peoples*. Garden City, NY: Anchor/ Doubleday.

Melton, J. Gordon. 1995. "Wither the New Age?" In *America's Alternative Religions*, Timothy Miller (ed.), pp. 347–352. Albany, NY: SUNY Press.

Menocal, María Rosa. 2002. *The Ornament of the World: How Muslims, Jews, and Christians Created a Culture of Tolerance in Medieval Spain*. New York: Little Brown.

Mosack, Katie, Mary Ann Abbott, Merrill Singer, Margaret Weeks, and Lucy Rohena. 2005. "If I Didn't Have HIV I'd Be Dead Now: Illness Narratives of Drug Users Living with HIV/AIDS." *Qualitative Health Research* 15(5): 586–605.

Murdock, George Peter. 1980. *Theories of Illness: A World Survey*. Pittsburgh: University of Pittsburgh Press.

Murphy, Joseph M. 1993. *Santería: African Spirits in America*. Boston: Beacon Press.

Murphy, Joseph M. 1995. "Santería and Vodou in the United States." In *America's Alternative Religions*, Timothy Miller (ed.), pp. 291–296. Albany: State University of New York Press.

Murray, Christopher J. L. and Alan D. Lopez. 1996. *Global Burden of Disease*. Boston: Harvard University Press (for WHO and World Bank).

Nichter, Mark (Ed.). 1992. *Anthropological Approaches to the Study of Ethnomedicine*. Amsterdam: Gordon and Breach Science Publishers.

Notestein, Frank W. 1945. "Population—The Long View." In *Food for the World*, Theodore W. Schultz (ed.), pp. 36–39. Chicago: University of Chicago Press.

Nuckolls, Charles W. 1992. "Deciding How to Decide: Possession-Mediumship in Jalari Divination." In *Anthropological Approaches to the Study of Ethnomedicine*, Mark Nichter (ed.), pp. 75–100. Amsterdam: Gordon and Breach Science Publishers.

O'Connor, Bonnie Blair. 1995. *Alternative Medicine and the Health Professions*. Philadelphia: University of Pennsylvania Press.

Olmos, Margarite Fernandez and Lizabeth Paravisini-Gebert (Eds.). 1997. *Sacred Possessions: Vodou, Santería, Obeah and the Caribbean*. New Brunswick, NJ: Rutgers University Press

Omran, A. K. 1971. "The Epidemiologic Transition: A Theory of the Epidemiology of Population Change." *Milbank Memorial Fund Quarterly* 49(4): 509–538.

Ohnuki-Tierney, Emiko. 1984. *Illness and Culture in Contemporary Japan: An Anthropological View*. Cambridge: Press Syndicate of the University of Cambridge.

Parsons, Claire D. F. (Ed.). 1985. *Healing Practices in the South Pacific*. Honolulu: The Institute for Polynesian Studies, University of Hawaii Press.

Parsons, Talcott. 1951. *The Social System*. New York: Free Press.

Population Reference Bureau. 2006. *2006 World Population Data Sheet*. Washington, DC: Author.

Quinlan, Marsha B. 2004. *From the Bush: The Front Line of Health Care in a Caribbean Village*. Belmont, CA: Wadsworth.

Reid, Janice. 1983. *Sorcerers and Healing Spirits: Continuity and Change in an Aboriginal Medical System*. Canberra: Australian National University Press.

Rivers, W. H. R. 1924. *Medicine, Magic, and Religion*. New York: Harcourt Brace.

Robarchek, Clayton and Carole Robarchek. 1998. *Waorani: The Contexts of Violence and War*. New York: Harcourt Brace.

Roberts, Charlotte and Keith Manchester. 2005. *The Archaeology of Disease*. Third Edition. Ithaca, NY: Cornell University Press.

Rubel, Arthur J. 1964. "The Epidemiology of a Folk Illness: Susto in Hispanic America." *American Ethnology* 3:268–283.

Rubel, Arthur J. and Michael R. Haas. 1996. "Ethnomedicine." In *Medical Anthropology: Contemporary Theory and Method*, Carolyn E. Sargent and Thomas M. Johnson (eds.), pp. 113–130. New York: Praeger.

Salguero, C. Pierce. 2003. *A Thai Herbal: Traditional Recipes for Health and Harmony*. Forres, Scotland: Findhorn Press.

Sargent, Carolyn F. and Thomas M. Johnson (Eds.). 1996. *Medical Anthropology: Contemporary Theory and Method*. Westport, CT: Praeger.

Scheper-Hughes, Nancy and Margaret M. Lock. 1987. "The Mindful Body: A Prolegomenon to Future Work in Medical Anthropology." *Medical Anthropology Quarterly* 1(1): 6–41.

Schoeppflin, Rennie B. 1988. Christian Science Healing in America. In *Other Healers. Unorthodox Medicine in America*, Norman Gevitz (ed.), pp. 192–214. Baltimore: The Johns Hopkins University Press.

Scrimshaw, Susan C. 2001. "Culture, Behavior, and Health." In *International Public Health: Diseases, Programs, Systems, and Policies*, Michael H. Merson, Robert E. Black, and Anne J. Mills (eds.), pp. 53–78. Gaithersgurg, MD: Aspen.

Selye, Hans. 1956. *The Stress of Life*. New York: McGraw-Hill.

Selye, Hans. 1976. *Stress in Health and Disease*. Boston: Butterworths.

Sharma, Ursula. 1992. *Complementary Medicine Today: Practitioners and Patients*. London and New York: Tavistock/Routledge.

Sheldon, Frances. 1998. "Bereavement. (ABC of Palliative Care)." *British Medical Journal* (February 7), 5 pages (online article).

Sierpina, Victor S. and Moshe A. Frenkel. 2005. "Acupuncture: A Clinical Review." *Southern Medical Journal* 98(3): 330–337.

Simons, Ronald C. and Charles C. Hughes (Eds.). 1985. *The Culture-Bound Syndromes: Folk Illnesses of Psychiatric and Anthropological Interest*. Dordrecht: D. Reidel.

Simons, Ronald C. 2001. "Introduction to Culture-Bound Syndromes." *Psychiatric Times* 18(11) (November) http://www.psychiatrictimes.com/p011163.html (accessed 1/16/06).

Singer Merrill. 1996. "A Dose of Drugs, a Touch of Violence, a Case of AIDS: Conceptualizing the SAVA Syndemic." *Free Inquiry* 24(2): 99–110.

Singer, Merrill. 2004. "Tobacco Use in Medical Anthropological Perspective." In *Encyclopedia of Medical Anthropology: Health and Illness in the World's Cultures*, Carol Ember and Melvin Ember, (eds.), pp. 518–527. New York: Kluwer.

Singer, Merrill. 2007. Ecosyndemics: Global Warming and the Coming Plagues of the 21st Century. Paper prepared for presentation at the Wenner-Gren Conference: Plagues: Models and Metaphors in the Human "Struggle with Disease" in October 2007.

Singer, Merrill and Scott Clair. 2003. "Syndemics and Public health: Reconceptualizing Disease in Bio-Social Context." *Medical Anthropology Quarterly* 17(4): 423–441.

Singer, Merrill, Lani Davison, and Gina Gerdes. 1988. "Culture, Critical Theory, and Reproductive Illness Behavior in Haiti." *Medical Anthropology Quarterly* 2(4): 370–385.

Singer, Merrill, Pamela I. Erickson, Louise Badiane, Rosemary Diaz, Dugeidy Ortiz, Traci Abraham, and Anna Marie Nicolaysen. 2006. "Syndemics, Sex and the City: Understanding Sexually Transmitted Diseases in Social and Cultural Context." *Social Science and Medicine* 63:2010–2021.

Singer, Merrill and Roberto Garcia. 1989. "Becoming a Puerto Rican Espiritista: Life History of a Female Healer." In *Women as Healers*, Carol Shepherd McClain (ed.), pp. 157–185. New Brunswick, NJ: Rutgers University Press.

Snow, Loudell F. 1993. *Walkin' Over Medicine*. Boulder, CO: Westview Press.

Sobo, Elisa J. 1992. "'Unclean Deeds': Menstrual Taboos and Binding 'Ties' in Rural Jamaica." In *Anthropological Approaches to the Study of Ethnomedicine*, Mark Nichter (ed.), pp. 101–126. Amsterdam: Gordon and Breach Science Publishers.

Starr, Paul 1982. *The Social Transformation of American Medicine.* San Francisco: Basic Books.

Strassmann, Beverly I. 1999. "Menstrual Synchrony Pheromones: Cause for Doubt." *Human Reproduction* 14(3): 579–580.

Sternberg, Esther M. 1997. "Emotions and Disease: From Balance of Humors to Balance of Molecules." *Nature Medicine* 3(3): 264–267.

Sternberg, Esther M. 2002. "Walter B. Cannon and 'Voodoo Death': A Perspective from 60 Years On." *American Journal of Public Health* 92(10): 1564–1565.

Stokols, Daniel. 2000. "Social Ecology and Behavioral Medicine: Implications for Training, Practice, and Policy." *Behavioral Medicine* 26(3): 129–138. https://vpn.uconn.edu/ehost/detail,DanaInfo=web.ebscohost.com+?vid=2 &hid=103&sid=b817d716-3bcb-40eb-8651-b66159aacb07%40session mgr106 (accessed on line through University of Connecticut Library in HTML format on 2/21/07, pp. 1–14).

Thomas, K. B. 1994. "The Placebo in General Practice." *The Lancet* 344(8929): 1066–1067.

Torres, Eliseo "Cheo" with Timothy L. Sawyer, Jr. 2005. *Curandero: A Life in Mexican Folk Healing.* Albuquerque: University of New Mexico Press.

University of California Extension Media Center (UCEMC). 1963. *Pomo Shaman* (CB2895), Black and White/Monochrome; sound; 22 minutes.

Voeks, Robert. 1993. "African Medicine and Magic in the Americas." *Geographical Review* 83(1): 66–78.

Voeks, Robert A. 1997. *Sacred Leaves of Candomblé: African Magic, Medicine, and Religion in Brazil.* Austin: University of Texas Press.

Waterhouse, Andrew L. 1995. "Wine and Heart Disease." *Chemistry & Industry* 1 (May): 338–341.

Webster, Jeanette I., Leonardo Tonelli, and Esther M. Sternberg. 2002. "Neuroendocrine Regulation of Immunity." *Annual Review of Immunology* 20:125–163.

Wedel, Johan 2004. *Santería Healing.* Gainseville: University of Florida Press.

Wein, Harrison. October, 2000. *Stress and Disease: New Perspectives.* NIH Office of Communications and Public Liaison. http://www.nih.gov/news/ WordonHealth/oct2000/story01.htm

Weller, Susan C. 1983. "New Data on Intracultural Variability: The Hot-Cold Concept of Medicine and Illness." *Human Organization* 42:249–257.

Wilce, James M., Jr. (Ed.). 2003. *Social and Cultural Lives of Immune Systems.* New York: Routledge.

Wilkinson, Richard and Michael Marmot (Eds.). 2003. *The Social Determinants of Health: The Solid Facts.* 2nd Edition. Copenhagen: World Health Organization, Regional Office for Europe.

World Health Organization, Alma-Ata. 1978. Primary Health Care: Report of the International Conference on Primary Health Care, Alma-Ata, USSR, 6–12 September 1978 ("Health for All" series, No. 1).

World Health Organization (WHO). 1993a. *Guidelines for the Primary Prevention of Mental, Neurological and Psychosocial Disorders: Principles for Primary Prevention.* Geneva: Division of Mental Health, World Health Organization.

World Health Organization (WHO). 1993b. Annex 2. *Culture-specific Disorders: ICD-10, Classification of Mental and Behavioral Disorders.* Geneva: World Health Organization, pp. 176–187.

World Health Organization (WHO). 2001. *Legal Status of Traditional Medicine and Complementary/Alternative Medicine: A Worldwide Review.* Geneva: World Health Organization.

World Health Organization (WHO). 2002a. *WHO Traditional Medicine Strategy 2002–2005.* Geneva: World Health Organization.

World Health Organization (WHO). 2002b. *World Report on Violence and Health: Summary.* Geneva: World Health Organization.

Yap, Pow M. 1965. "Koro—A Culture-bound Depersonalization Syndrome." *British Journal of Psychiatry* 3:43–50.

Yap, Pow M. 1969a. "Classification of the Culture-bound Reactive Syndromes." *Far East Medical Journal* 7:219–225.

Yap, Pow M. 1969b. "The Culture-bound Reactive Syndromes." In *Mental Health Research in Asia and the Pacific*, William Caudill and Tsung-yi Lin (eds.), pp. 33–53. Honolulu: East-West Center Press,

Young, Allan. 1982. "The Anthropologies of Illness and Sickness." *Annual Review of Anthropology* 11:257–285.

Young, James Clay and Linda C. Garro. 1994 [1981]. *Medical Choice in a Mexican Village.* Long Grove, IL: Waveland Press.

Zimmerman, Michael R. 2004. "Paleopathology and the Study of Ancient Remains." In *Encyclopedia of Medical Anthropology, Health and Illness in the Worlds Cultures, Volume 1: Topics*, Carol R. Ember and Melvin Ember (eds.), pp. 49–58. New York: Kluwer.

Index